A Special CRM Collection

Exciting Crew Resource Management Topics

Examples From Aviation and Emergency Medicine

Volume 1

Eva-Maria Schottdorf

A Special CRM Collection

Exciting Crew Resource Management Topics
Examples From Aviation and Emergency Medicine

Volume 1

Eva-Maria Schottdorf

Communicatio optima

Munich

Correspondence Address of the Author-Publisher
Eva-Maria Schottdorf MD MSc
Communicatio optima
Alte Hopfenpost
Hopfenstraße 8
80335 Munich
Germany
Email: service@communicatio-optima.com
Website: https://www.communicatio-optima.com

Availability of the Book and Discounts on Bulk Orders
This book is sold from the publisher's website and available from most online booksellers. Professional organisations who order directly from the publisher will receive a sizable discount on bulk orders. For more information, please use the aforementioned contact details.

Design and Proofreading
Cover Design: Schottdorf EM
Cover Photograph: Schottdorf EM
Layout and Figures: Schottdorf EM
Proofreader: Franziska Boldt

Bibliographical Information
The German National Library lists this publication in the German National Bibliography. Detailed bibliographic data can be accessed on the internet at:
https://www.dnb.de/DE/Home/home_node.html

Available Editions and Book Formats
1. English Edition as EBook 2024
ISBN 978-3-98925-005-5

1. English Edition as Print on Demand Book 2024
ISBN 978-3-98925-004-8

1. English Edition as 3D Flipbook 2024
ISBN 978-3-98925-008-6

1. German Edition as 3D Flipbook 2024
ISBN 978-3-98925-009-3

1. German Edition as EBook 2024
ISBN 978-3-98925-007-9

1. German Edition as Print on Demand Book 2024
ISBN 978-3-98925-006-2

"Always try to keep the number of landings you make
equal to the number of take-offs."

Anonymous

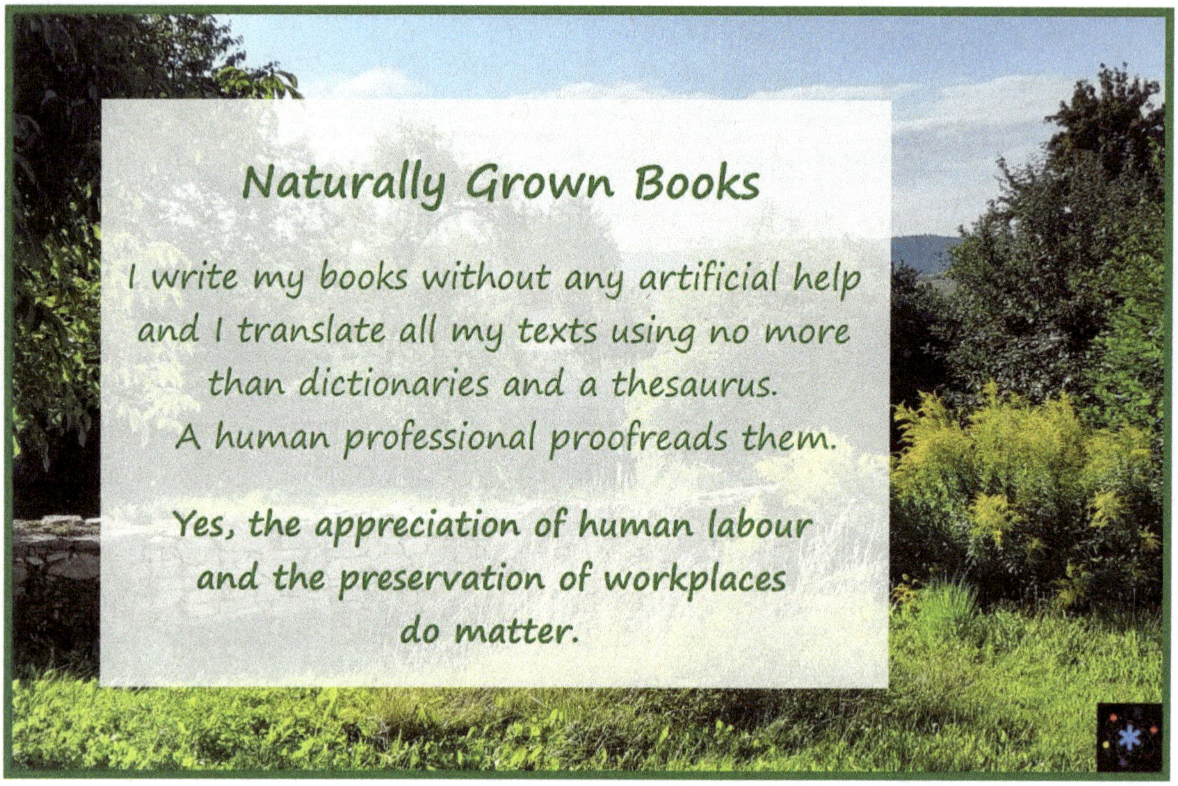
Naturally Grown Books
I write my books without any artificial help and I translate all my texts using no more than dictionaries and a thesaurus. A human professional proofreads them.
Yes, the appreciation of human labour and the preservation of workplaces do matter.

Preface to the Book Series "A Special CRM Collection"

Landing an aeroplane safely after every single take-off requires much knowledge, a variety of skills, and the right attitude. What other resources do the pilots and their cabin crews have at their disposal to fulfil this expectation, which every passenger has as a matter of course?

The crew resource management themes, which we will explore together in this book series, will be taken from the entire subject area. All the topics will be as instructive as they will be beneficial. Some of them will be less known, whilst others will be about particularly interesting cases of all sorts. In addition, we will examine a few of the major incidents in aviation, as well as air accidents, paying close attention to what has been learned from the meticulous investigation of these dangerous and in some cases tragic events.

We will unveil how CRM is used today in aviation, where it originated, as well as in medicine, where it is continuously introduced into more and more specialty fields. For this, we will use many examples from both lines of business. In addition, the principles applied in CRM are of great value in many professions in which teamwork and the avoidance of momentous mistakes play a decisive role. Hence, I would like to invite you to consider how you would apply what you have just read at your workplace. To facilitate this, I will include short "Pause and Think" sections as an opportunity for you to take your time and reflect before reading on.

This book series about important CRM topics is not a detailed classic textbook. Rather, its themes will be presented in separate chapters for you to read independently from one another. You can enjoy them without any preexisting CRM knowledge, or, if you are a professional who has used CRM already, as a short refreshment of what you have already learned.

Each volume will comprise twelve chapters. The content of each one has initially served as a blog article on my website, where I publish a new one every month. As these original articles represent a whole year, you will find a Christmas chapter at the end, which adds to the more relaxed atmosphere in this book series. At the same time, I have updated the information where needed and supported it with an array of didactic features. You can find a compilation of those under "The Features in This Book", starting at page 3. I hope to see you in the main part of the book!

Eva-Maria Schottdorf

Munich, August 2023

Preface to Volume 1 of the Special CRM Collection

Here, I will briefly outline for you, what topics you will find in this first volume. We will start off with a crucial topic, the importance of which is often overlooked: how to give and receive praise. Unfortunately, praise does not belong to the wide variety of CRM principles (yet). In the first chapter, we will elucidate what type of praise really helps us to grow as professionals.

Just as important as praise is the analysis of brilliant achievements. Why? We will look at this in-depth in the second chapter. You might already have heard about knowledge, skills, and attitude. We will explore these three areas of learning in the third chapter. Which of these is the hardest to change and optimise? After so much input, two chapters will be dedicated to the different types of stress and how to deal with them successfully.

What happened on Qantas Flight 32 in November 2010? Whether you are familiar with this incident or not, does not matter at all. In chapter six, we will examine the events step by step, and see how truly professional pilots showed admirable courage and real leadership and teamwork in order to combine all their knowledge and skills to counteract the myriad of problems they were facing. It is almost astounding, how much CRM we will detect there.

What is the difference between threats and errors? How are they interrelated? What causes an undesired aircraft state (UAS)? Find out in chapter seven, where you will also learn how to deal with threats and errors in your profession successfully.

The error chain is not the chain of events. In chapter eight, we will discover what it is and how we can break its links using CRM principles. In chapter nine, we will apply the error chain to the most devastating air accident in the history of civil aviation.

What is just culture? We will disclose the secret in chapter ten and learn why this fundamental concept was developed. In chapter eleven, we will place just culture in the crucial area of expertise to which it belongs.

Finally, we will have deserved some relaxing moments. Why not join the industrious bakers in the pre-Christmas kitchen? Moreover, would it not be nice to apply some of our CRM knowledge, which we have acquired so eagerly? Yes, it will be fun, and the results will be great!

Eva-Maria Schottdorf

Munich, August 2023

Acknowledgements

I thank my proofreader, Franziska Boldt, for her great work.

I started writing my blog in January 2021. Right from the start, I had eager readers who provided me with invaluable comments and suggestions, amongst them Beate Ebel, Christina Gilg, and Christine Perner-Neidhardt. Thank you so much for your keen interest and continued support. You helped me greatly to lay the foundation for this book series.

From the very beginning of my education as a seminar trainer and later an author-publisher, I have worked closely together with Christine Perner-Neidhardt, who is a successful business owner herself. Our ongoing discussions about many business aspects, including webdesign, sparked some of my most important ideas. Speaking of design, I would like to thank my dear friend Karen Richter, a brilliant graphic designer, for her precious tips concerning so many different issues in this field.

Crew resource management has fascinated me ever since I was introduced to it. I am interested in all of its topics, especially in how it is used in aviation. To this day, I am really grateful to my wonderful CRM trainers, Anne Sølvsteen and Jesper Høyer Rasmussen, at NaviMinds in Copenhagen, Denmark, who are both truly seasoned aviation professionals. They not only taught me CRM comprehensively but also really inspired my teaching.

As a prehospital emergency physician, I have worked with many a great team over the years. I would like to thank all of them not only for their great collaboration, using CRM, but also for their true camaraderie.

Last but not least, I thank my family and close friends for their human warmth and companionship, but also for our in-depth discussions, in which we make one another aware of so many important aspects in life. It is even more important that these discussions show our sincere interest in one another, which is priceless.

Table of Contents

Table of Contents

Table of Contents

Table of Contents

List of Figures

List of Tables

List of Abbreviations

ATC	air traffic control
ATSB	Australian Transport Safety Bureau
CAA	civil aviation authority
CFIT	controlled flight into terrain
CRM	crew resource management
EASA	European Union Aviation Safety Agency
ECAM	electronic centralised aircraft monitor
EMS	emergency medical service
ETA	estimated arrival time
FAA	Federal Aviation Administration
FAST	face, arms, speech, time
FORDEC	facts, options, risks, decision, execution, check
HF	human factors
KLM	Koninklijke Luchtvaart Maatschappij N.V., Royal Aviation Company Plc.
ICAO	International Civil Aviation Organization
IATA	International Air Transport Association
LOSA	line operation safety audit
MRM	maintenance resource management
NTSB	National Transportation Safety Board
Pan Am	Pan American World Airways
PF	pilot flying
PM	pilot monitoring
SMS	safety management system
SOP	standard operating procedure
TDODAR	time, diagnose, options, decide, act/assign, review
TEM	threat and error management
UAS	undesired aircraft state
UERF	uncontained engine rotor failure
VHF	very high frequency
YT	YouTube

The Features in This Book

The Beginning of a New Chapter

In order to make it as convenient as possible for you, each chapter will start with a small table of contents containing all second-level headings. There will also be a small introduction.

The Various Text Boxes

You will encounter six types of text boxes as described below:

Pause and Think

These will contain an opportunity to reflect on a certain issue in relation to your work or what you expect to read in the following sections. It is by no means an assessment of any sort, so don't worry.

Remember

Concise sentences will make it easy for you to remember important concepts and items of CRM.

Top Tips and Secrets

The top tips will help with difficult tasks, whereas the secrets will be from my own work experience.

Pitfalls and How to Avoid Them

In these text boxes, I will point out common pitfalls to you and show you how can navigate around them successfully.

The 15 CRM Key Points

In the second volume of this series, I will introduce you to the 15 CRM Key Points by Rall and Gaba. We will occupy ourselves in-depth with them in the CRM Book Series.

The Comprehensive Summary of Each Chapter

The summary will contain all the important key messages of a chapter compiled in a handy list.

Additional Material

Figures and Tables

There will be tables and figures, as you might have seen in case you went through the respective lists above. Speaking of lists, some lists will also be included in the text, containing the facts for you to read at a glance.

Handy Cheat Sheets

At the end of each volume, you will find two cheat sheets, on which a wealth of information on a relevant topic is compiled. On the first cheat sheet of this volume, I will provide you with a step by step guide on how to integrate what you have just read into your own work processes. On the second one, I will summarise important information on the speak up which you can use at your workplace.

Separate Glossaries

I have included separate glossaries for aviation, CRM, and medical terms so that you can concentrate on one area of knowledge as you look up a certain concept or definition.

The Index

The index rounds off this book. There, you will only find the page on which a term is explained so that you obtain a maximum of information in one go.

After so much introduction, let us delve into the fascinating world of crew resource management right away!

1

1. Real Praise Works Miracles

These Contents Are Waiting for You in the First Chapter

As a start into this this Special CRM Collection, we will explore an important theme, which is often overlooked, not only when practising crew resource management but also in our daily lives. We will highlight, what sincere praise is and what we can achieve when we accustom ourselves not only to give but also to receive such a recognition. We will also discover that there are different types of praise. Which one is most helpful?

1.1. Before We Really Get Started

Pause and Think

Can you say off the top of your head when you received praise lately?

Here, we will shed light on the effects of praise that not only spur us on to new accomplishments, but also lets us understand why we have achieved something. We will not take a closer look at constructive feedback. Such feedback is something positive, because it helps us to learn, to mend our weaknesses, and to correct our mistakes. The following chapter might provide food for thought for all of us. It is not intended to be a scientific paper.

1.2. The Status Quo in Our Daily Lives

When we start looking at praise honestly, what do our everyday lives look like many a time at work and especially in private? Don't you instantly remember situations in which your masterpieces, after you had invested much time and effort, have been taken for granted? What do you feel if this is the norm and a "no criticism is praise enough" culture prevails? Haven't we ourselves already reacted to our fellow human beings´ superb achievements with a mere and short "thank you" before?

At this point, a huge praise to all of you who know how to praise wisely at the right time.

1.3. How to Accept and Enjoy Praise

We know that some of us do not feel comfortable when having to accept praise. The ones concerned feel embarrassed when receiving it, especially in front of others. They then tend to downplay their achievements. Why is that? What do we accomplish if we encourage these people among us to acknowledge their achievements for themselves?

If we develop a positive view of ourselves and not only recognise our mistakes, we are able to optimise our poise and unfold our skills to their fullest potential. Of course, we should thereby aim at assessing our achievements and our abilities realistically and keep our feet on the ground.

1.4. What to Praise

As Allison Master explains in her article „Praise That Makes Learners More Resilient" (1) there is praise for personal traits, for instance, a great talent for drawing, and praise for the process which we applied in order to achieve something.

Naturally, we are delighted by praise for a positive trait. However, we cannot control a mere trait in the same way we can control a process. We can control our strategies, though, as well as our problem solving skills, and how we gather and use information. Praise for one of these helps us to understand why we have been successful.

1.5. How We Draw Strength From Praise if Something Has Gone Wrong

Praise that is attached to a process even helps us when we were not able to complete a task as intended. As opposed to praise, which we receive for one of our traits, it helps us to recognise that we do not have to question ourselves in general if something has gone wrong. We are not generally incapable of completing the task successfully.

Rather, we do have the necessary resources in ourselves and only have to reconsider our approach. Did we choose the right strategy? Did we work hard enough? Did we use the appropriate knowledge and information? Thus, we are able to determine what we need to change in order to obtain the desired result next time.

1.6. Further Positive Aspects of Praise

Generally speaking, praise for our efforts along the way can optimise an outcome, because it motivates us. If it is praise for the process we are using, we know that we can trust our course of action. Praise for something we have achieved can spur us on to push ourselves even more and to set ourselves new goals taking advantage of the confidence we have gained.

1.7. A Training Course, One Detail, and Its Enormous Impact

I became aware (again) of the — often underestimated — importance of judicious praise during my CRM Trainer Course in Copenhagen in 2020.

Right from the start, it was part of the course concept to be prepared to be praised and to praise, no matter whether you were a participant or a trainer. Already in the invitation letter, an entire item was dedicated solely to this aspect. In addition, it attracted attention that it was not about superficialness, but honest recognition of great performances, which, of course, had to be delivered and were delivered by everyone involved.

1.8. Let's Integrate Praise Into Our Daily Routine

As the praise in Copenhagen has quickened the atmosphere of our training course so constructively, I am convinced that appropriate praise at the right time is absolutely beneficial. We should embrace practising the art of praising. Last but not least, I want to encourage you not only to be able to praise sincerely, but also to accept and enjoy such a recognition.

1.9. The Comprehensive Summary of Chapter 1

Giving praise for a process at the right time is crucially important and beneficial.

- praising is quite often not a natural part of our daily routine or at our workplace
- some people feel ashamed when being praised publicly; they downplay their achievements
- there are two types of praise, for a trait or for a process we have used
- the latter helps us to understand why we have been successful
- praise for a process even helps us when something went wrong
- sincere praise for a task well done quickens the atmosphere enhances our motivation
- we should learn not only to give sincere praise but also to enjoy it

1.10. In the Next Chapter You Will Learn...

... why our successes want to be analysed as well.

1.11. Reference

1) Allison Master (2015) Praise That Makes Learners More Resilient. Student Experience Research Network, https://studentexperiencenetwork.org/wp-content/uploads/2015/09/Praise-That-Makes-Learners-More-Reslient.pdf. Most recently accessed: July 15th, 2023

2

2. Our Successes Want to Be Analysed, Too

These Contents Are Waiting for You in the Second Chapter

Finally, after years of hard work and many team training sessions, we deliver a perfect piece of teamwork in a scenario during such a session. As with praise, which may be scarce at some workplaces, major successes may not be acknowledged and analysed appropriately during the debriefing which follows the scenario. Why is that? Furthermore, what do we gain if we elaborate carefully why we achieved our success? Let us find out on the following pages.

2.1. We Start With a Team Training

Pause and Think

Have you ever taken part in a practical team training focusing on the principles of crew resource management? Or in any other type of team training? Or have you simply got a lot of experience from your daily team work?

2.1.1. What the Training Is Like

For all of you who have not experienced a CRM training yet, we will look at a medical training scenario as an example. That way, we can compile step by step, how major successes are achieved. Furthermore, we will learn how to analyse and repeat them.

Let us imagine an emergency department where nurses and doctors treat a severely ill patient together. An actress mimes the patient. Instructors watch the team and pay particular attention to team-leading and teamwork. For example, they focus on communication and application of the CRM principles, such as the wise use of all resources and workload management.

2.1.2. The Road to Brilliant Coups Is Rocky

As no one is born a master, even this professional and experienced team makes some mistakes. For instance, pieces of information are lost, and relevant announcements, such as blood values, go unnoticed. Consequently, necessary conclusions are not drawn. Sometimes, uncertainty about workload management occurs. Therefore, some tasks are not performed, whilst others are done redundantly, for instance, the preparation of a medical procedure.

Ideally, all resources are used, including all team members′ efforts, every piece of information, and technical equipment. As you can imagine, in a complex situation, this is not always easily accomplished at the right time.

Remember

The aim of CRM is that team members discover errors early and correct them before these errors have any impact on their patients.

2.2. We Work Towards Successes During the Debriefing Session

During the debriefing session, the instructors and the team discuss the issues, which the members can still improve. When we are taking part in a debriefing session ourselves, we often recognise immediately where we went wrong. Small mistakes may appear so large that great achievements seem to be marginal in comparison. In addition, videotapes of the scenario are sometimes shown. This may feel embarrassing as we seldom think that we are shown in the most favourable manner. Thus, a debriefing session following a training scenario is not the most relaxing experience, no matter how much the instructors strive to create a pleasant and constructive atmosphere.

Remember

We can only improve by analysing our mistakes and their underlying causes together.

2.3. Finally, We Achieve a Brilliant Coup

Having gone through many scenarios and debriefing sessions, one day we perform THE scenario as a team. We carry out everything perfectly, from communication to fulfilling the task successfully. According to our experience, such a successful scenario is seldom analysed in-depth during the debriefing session, either because the team is well-known for being great, or it has simply performed everything perfectly this time.

Pitfall

So, what should we talk about? Let us rather spend our time analysing scenarios that require improvement.

However, why were we so successful as a team in this case? Was it by chance? Or are we a real dream team that owns a secret recipe for success?

Remember

In order to find out what the cause of our success is, we need to analyse our perfectly performed scenarios in the same way as the ones we have to improve.

2.4. We Analyse Our Brilliant Coup

Exemplarily, we will shed light on the topics already mentioned above, communication, workload management, and the use of resources. We will also discover how the CRM principles as such help us to perform the task.

2.4.1. Communication Without Loss of Information

Safe and Effective Communication

As team members we have delivered clear messages making sure that the others listened to them actively and acted accordingly.

Closed Communication Loops

Closed communication loops play a major role in communication without loss of information. When we receive a message, we repeat what has been said. Using this type of feedback together with the sender, we ensure that the content of the message came across as intended. Besides, we have the opportunity to question a message.

Speak up

Every team member is allowed to speak up at any time. Thus, we guarantee that every team member's possible concerns are heard and evaluated. If we explore such concerns and take action where necessary, we avoid making — potentially momentous — mistakes.

2.4.2. Wisely and Clearly Communicated Workload Management

Everyone was adequately busy, no one had too much or too little to do at any time. The tasks matched the respective knowledge and the skills accordingly and did not overstrech anyone.

Our team leader always had a good overview over all the tasks. He or she distributed them and received confirmation once they were finished. Those who had too many or too difficult tasks let the team leader know, as did the ones who were available to take on new jobs.

2.4.3. Use of All Available Resources

As mentioned in the preceding paragraph, each of us was involved in the teamwork at all times. Furthermore, we made use of all available pieces of information and our technical resources.

2.5. Now We Can Repeat Our Major Success

If we analyse our in this case perfect use of the CRM principles, we will find out why our teamwork went smoothly and why we were able to perform our task safely and in a structured manner.

Top Tip

If we understand why we were successful, we know that our success was not due to luck. Rather, we know that we are able to repeat our brilliant coup and even build on it.

2.6. We Transfer Major Successes From Team Training Into Daily Life

After having worked so hard during team training, we should transfer the results of the analysis of our brilliant coups from CRM training into different areas of our routine work. The entire cycle from the scenario to this crucial step is depicted in Figure 1.

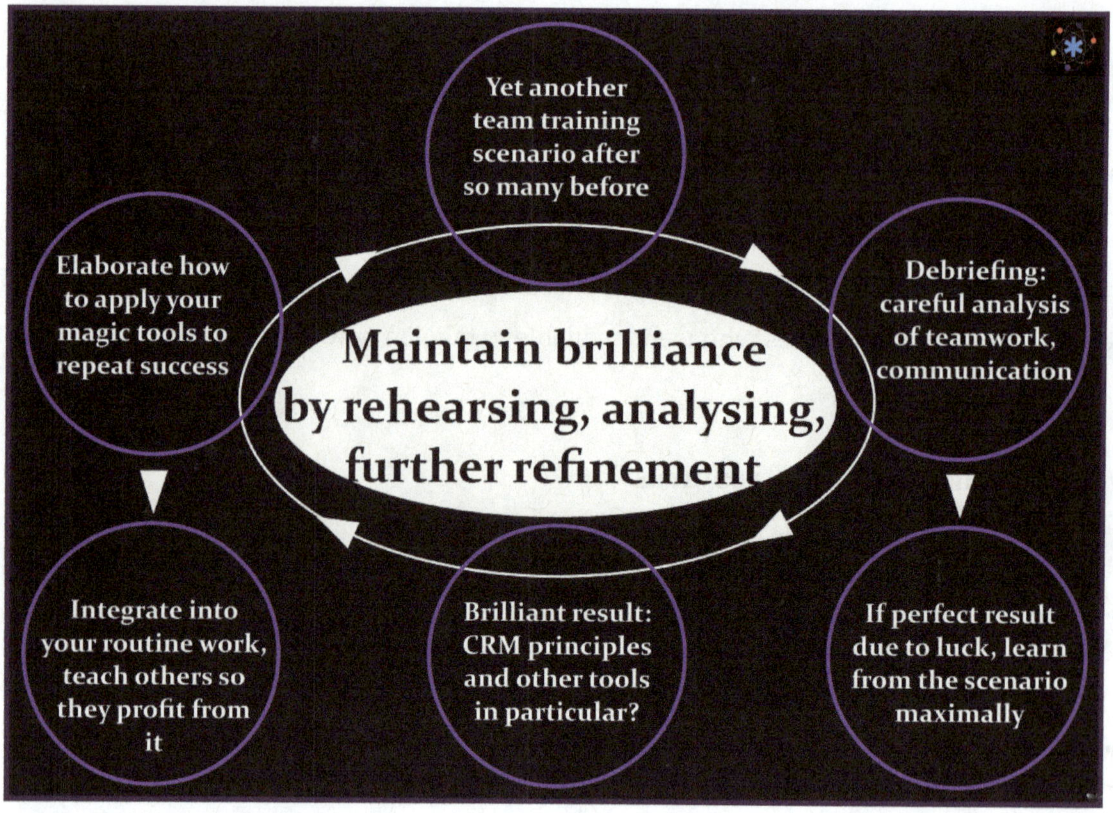

Figure 1 Analysis of brilliant coups

Pause and Think

What situations, which you have mastered superbly together with others, do you remember?

What was the secret of your success?

2.7. The Comprehensive Summary of Chapter 2

Only by analysing brilliant pieces of teamwork can we understand the cause of our success.

- perfect teamwork is the result of hard work and many team training sessions
- the need to analyse a superbly performed scenario is often overlooked
- we can only answer the question why we have been successful if we scrutinise brilliant work

2.8. Knowledge, Skills, and Attitude Ahead

We apply knowledge, skills, and the right attitude during our teamwork. Which of these three essential ingredients is the most difficult one to optimise?

3

3. Knowledge, Skills, and Attitude

These Contents Are Waiting for You in the Third Chapter

Knowledge, skills, and attitude are the three areas of learning. In this chapter, we will unveil which of the three is the most difficult one to optimise and why. Of course, we will also highlight how we can achieve the optimisation nonetheless, using the introduction of CRM as an example.

3.1. First of All, a Fancy Cake Is Being Baked

Three friends are baking a fancy cake for the birthday party to which they are invited that night. They know the ingredients, and in which order they have to mix them into the dough. They know when they have to heat the oven and how long the baking time will be. They know when they have to prepare the filling and when to spread it, after the cake has cooled down. They are able to transfer the cake onto the wire rack for cooling. They cut the cake into perfect cake slices and spread the filling evenly on all of them. Finally, they decorate their fancy cake with aptness and finesse. To leave the landlady's kitchen tidied up perfectly and spotlessly clean, is a point of honour.

Knowledge, skills, and attitude — you have certainly noticed, where the three of them have employed which component beneficially in their teamwork. Additionally, we understand that knowledge, skills, and attitude are vital in any kind of teamwork.

3.2. Where Do Our Knowledge, Skills, and Attitude Come From?

3.2.1. Knowledge

Sometimes, for example during spare time activities, we acquire knowledge playfully. At other times, we have to cram with diligence and volition until we have a command of the subject. Sometimes, an exam forces us to study, and sometimes we realise ourselves that we need the respective knowledge. It certainly helps us to connect the new knowledge with what we already know or to reflect on how we are going to use it.

3.2.2. Skills

Everywhere in our lives we face practical skills, which we want to or have to be able to do. It does not matter whether we look our three friends in the kitchen mentioned above over their shoulders, or do some DIY, play a sport, or learn medical examination techniques. We have to practise these skills until we are able to carry them out as required or until we meet our own expectations. Sometimes, we may become frustrated, but we carry on.

3.2.3. Attitude

We bring our attitude to our teamwork alongside our knowledge and skills. An attitude is an opinion, a thought, or a feeling, we have about people, situations, or other things. It influences our behaviour as well as that of others, whilst working together.

Pause and Think

Are we always conscious of our attitude? From where have we got it? Is it constructive or can we mend anything?

If we want to optimise it, we need to recognise the necessity to do so in the first place. Sometimes, it is not as apparent as the necessity to acquire knowledge and skills.

Remember

Therefore, and due to the role traditions play, it is most difficult to change our attitude. Only with our attitude we establish the cooperative and constructive atmosphere in our teamwork, in which we use our knowledge and skills to the fullest.

Now, we dare to approach this most demanding of the three areas of learning, knowledge, skills, and attitude. In the following paragraphs, we will elaborate how to perfect our attitude, using CRM as an example.

3.3. We Work on Our Attitude

3.3.1. The Attitude Towards Bosses and Subordinates in the Past

In aviation, until the beginning of the 1970s, pilots were seen as indisputable heroes, who made the decisions. The other members in the cockpit assisted and were mostly not actively involved in the decision-making process. Also in healthcare, team members did frequently not dare to speak up, even if they had discovered an error. Hence, it was the widespread attitude in those times that bosses in different lines of business were not to be questioned.

However, too many air disasters occurred, claiming lives almost every time. As is commonly known, the worst disaster in aviation to date has been the collision of two jumbo jets on the runway on the island of Tenerife in March 1977.

3.3.2. Questioning Attitude and Recognising the Necessity to Change

All air disasters are painstakingly examined, in order to find the cause, but also to establish how the mistakes discovered can be prevented in the future. One of the results, also concerning the crash in Tenerife (1), was the discovery that error chains lead to accidents. Human error, especially communication errors, plays the main role in more than 70% of such catastrophes.

Consequently, crew resource management was established. It includes a novel view on the roles in a team. Besides, one had recognised the necessity to reconsider the attitude towards the relationship between a boss and his or her subordinates. This is evident in CRM concepts, such as the speak up and closed communication loops.

3.3.3. The Cycle from Planning to Evaluation

If we want to change something, we need a cycle, which allows us to plan the change, to discuss the planned steps, and, finally, to put these steps into action. As we know, even well thought-out change processes never work according to plan. Thus, we try things out practically and evaluate our successes, as well as the room for improvement. Following that, we start the cycle anew based on our results (Figure 2).

However, does everyone agree to the intended change immediately? Even CRM met resistance as it was being developed. It was not established within one day, but in six generations (2), each of them with its own focus, starting in 1979.

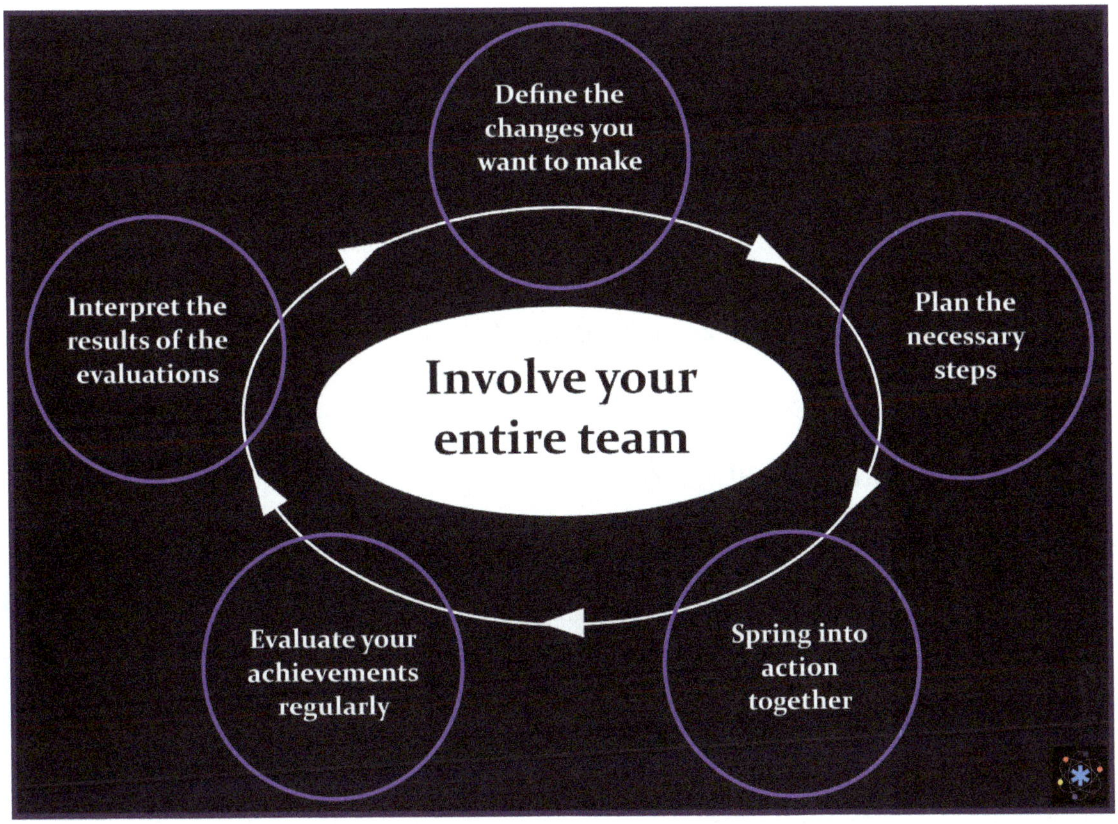

Figure 2 Working on our attitude

3.4. We Meet Obstacles and..... the Traditions

Pause and Think

Have you ever discussed attitudes with your team and worked on them?

If so, what difficulties have you encountered?

Such obstacles are nothing new, of course, and only human. Here, you find some of them summarised briefly:

- colleagues who are afraid of losing their current role or authority
- coworkers who cannot recognise the benefit of the project
- coworkers who are against it per se
- coworkers in any role, who are constructively critical — of course, they are not an obstacle in this spirit

- coworkers who are afraid not to be able to cope with the new requirements
- coworkers who see themselves taken by surprise and their plans completely disrupted
- coworkers who are afraid of more responsibility
- obstacles which you can name additionally

What shall we do with our traditions? How about renewing them where necessary and deliberately keeping tried and tested concepts that are still valuable?

3.5. We Overcome the Obstacles

Pause and Think

How have you managed to overcome obstacles on your way to changes so far?

As in every change management process, we come a long way if we bring everyone in early, state the reasons transparently, and invite constructive suggestions actively. As we move along, we should let everyone involved share their thoughts, opinions, and feelings.

Let us now look at possible ways to overcome the obstacles mentioned above:

- We should address the fear of losing one's role openly and discuss new responsibilities constructively.
- We should state the benefits transparently, preferably supported by scientific results. We should answer questions and meet doubt with open questions. We should prepare our answers. If we cannot give an answer, we should work it out and then come back to the person who asked.
- We should meet the ones who are against it with open questions in order to find out whether they can justify their scepticism.
- We should listen to the constructive critics, praise good suggestions and integrate those into the concept. If we cannot accept a suggestion, we should state the reason why.
- We should explore possible fears of new tasks and work out help and learning opportunities together.
- We should announce plans to change early and let the ones who need a precise plan take their time. Additionally, we should offer them the opportunity to support the planning process.

- Why does the fear of taking more responsibility exist? We should explore this together using open questions and discuss further education or a new role as necessary.
- Your additional solutions. We should always ask our team members if they have anything to add.

3.6. The Changed Attitude in CRM Helps to Detect Errors Early

3.6.1. The Changed Attitude

In a CRM team, everyone should contribute and his or her concerns or suggestions should be heard, regardless of his or her position in the team. Hence, today's attitude is different to the one from the 1970s mentioned above.

3.6.2. Using This Attitude, We Detect Mistakes Early

With our present-day attitude, all of us in the team use their knowledge and skills the best they can, applying the various CRM concepts. As is known, even when using CRM, we cannot avoid making mistakes one hundred percent.

Remember

However, with the help of the CRM concepts, we as a team discover errors as early as possible, before they cause any harm.

3.6.3. Let's Improve and... Celebrate Your Successes!

Whenever we change something, we should set ourselves measurable goals, document the results of our work and assess them. We should present our analyses to everyone involved transparently and improve together, what needs to be optimised.

Top Tip

Of course, we should celebrate our successes together as a team. We are explicitly allowed to praise our colleagues and motivate them to keep going. I wish you many opportunities to do so!

3.7. The Comprehensive Summary of Chapter 3

Three areas of learning: knowledge, skills, and attitude; the latter is most difficult to optimise.

- knowledge, skills, and attitude are important whenever we work as a team
- with our attitude we create the atmosphere in which we can fully use our knowledge and skills
- attitude is the hardest to ameliorate because of traditions and obstacles
- obstacles include: uncertainties concerning roles and abilities, disrupted plans
- we should include our entire team right from the start of the planned improvements
- we should set measurable goals and decide, how to measure progress towards them
- we should praise our team members and celebrate our successes together with them

3.8. The Next Chapter Is Not Meant to Be Stressful

We will elucidate, what different types of stress exist, and which of those we can use for great achievements. We will also highlight how to keep all other kinds of stress at bay, in order to master important CRM concepts, such as workload management, situational awareness, and decision-making, nonetheless.

3.9. References

1) ICAO Circular 153-AN/56, which contains:

1. Title page: Raad voor de Luchtvaart, Netherlands Aviation Safety Board, Final Report and Comments of the Netherlands Aviation Safety Board of the investigation into the accident with the collision of KLM flight 4805, Boeing 747-206B, PH-BUF, and Pan American flight 1736, Boeing 737-121, N736PA, at the Tenerife Airport, Spain, on 27 March 1977.

2. The Spanish Report (October 1978) Part 1 (The Investigation, page 22 = first page, and following) and Part 2 (Analysis and Conclusions, page 42 and following).

3. Comments of the State of Registry (Kingdom of The Netherlands), page 57 and following.

The ICAO Circular can be downloaded from: https://www.faasafety.gov/files/gslac/courses/content/232/1081/finaldutchreport.pdf, most recently accessed: July 23rd, 2023

Links to the Spanish Report in English Part 1 and 2:

http://www.project-tenerife.com/engels/PDF/Spanish_report.PDF, most recently accessed: July 29th, 2023

http://www.project-tenerife.com/engels/PDF/spanish_report2.PDF, most recently accessed: July 29th, 2023

2) Helmreich B (2006) Red Alert. World-renowned expert on human factors, Bob Helmreich, reviews the development of CRM since it was first introduced 25 years ago. Flight Safety Australia, September-October 2006. https://skybrary.aero/sites/default/files/bookshelf/1095.pdf, most recently accessed: July 20th, 2023

4

4. Stress, Management and Relevance in CRM — Part I

These Contents Are Waiting for You in the Fourth Chapter

Eustress, distress, hyperstress, hypostress, acute and chronic stress, but don't get stressed. We will elaborate step by step what causes all of these kinds of stress, what to use to our advantage and how to spot and counteract harmful stress. We will also start looking into how stress and CRM are interrelated.

4.1. We Start With Definitions in a Relaxed Manner

At the end of the day, there is still a lot of work left. Time, however, has run out once again. Too many tasks in too many areas of our lives demand our attention. Almost all of us recognise this. Will we ever get a chance to turn this situation around? Of course, we don't have a chance at all, but we will use it right now. Let us start.

In this chapter, we will deal with stress and take a look at why this topic is important in CRM in subchapter 4.8. For instance, stress influences important CRM components, such as workload management and decision-making. In the next chapter, we will take a closer look at the linkage and the interplay of stress and CRM principles. We will also elucidate, how CRM helps us to maintain an overview in stressful situations.

4.1.1. Defining Stress

Hans Selye initiated stress research. He defined stress as "the non-specific response of the body to any demand for change" (1). After we will have worked our way through the different types of stress step by step, you will find a summary of them and a selection of their causes, signs, and how to deal with them in Table 1 in subchapter 4.7.5.

4.1.2. Different Forms of Stress

We distinguish eustress and distress, as well as hyperstress and hypostress. Additionally, we speak of acute and chronic stress. "Eu" means beautiful, much, or good in ancient Greek. We will discuss this beneficial type of stress in subchapter 4.2. The opposite is distress, from the Latin verb "distringere", to draw apart, to hinder. Distress is the one that harms us.

We distinguish hyper- and hypostress. In ancient Greek "hyper" means beyond. Hyperstress is caused by too large a workload. The preposition "hypo" means under. Thus, hypostress is the consequence of too few challenges. We define stress as acute or chronic, depending on how long it lasts.

4.2. Eustress Helps Us to Perform Excellently

Pause and Think

What do you feel if you have to prepare an important presentation or a report for the board of directors? Or when you are planning to invite several guests to a grand dinner involving an exquisite set meal?

We all recognise such situations, which present a challenge to us and cause tension. Yet, we know that we will master this challenge if we take the right steps. We feel eustress. A certain amount of pressure, in the form of eustress, helps us to focus. We work stringently and concentratedly during our preparations, as well as during the actual performance. Eustress provides us with the extra amount of energy and creativity we need. We use it to achieve an excellent result.

4.3. Hyper- and Hypostress

4.3.1. Hyperstress

Hyperstress occurs if we have too much to do at once, if we haven't got enough time, and if these circumstances last for a longer period of time. Furthermore, we may pressure ourselves by imposing ourselves expectations we almost cannot fulfil. Hence, we will not be satisfied with some of the outcomes.

4.3.2. Hypostress

Hypostress occurs if there are too few challenges, concerning the amount of tasks, but also the level of difficulty. If we are in hypostress, our attention decreases, as does our drive with which we otherwise accomplish things swiftly and efficiently. Moreover, we may become complacent, as our performance horizon narrows, and our awareness of our talents dwindles when we lack challenges. Frustration, boredom and the feeling not being needed may arise as well, minimising our drive and motivation further.

4.4. Distress Exhausts Us

This unpleasant type of stress is caused by demands that exceed our capacities. In addition, incisive events in our lives, such as losing a job, losing a loved one, or a divorce, distress us.

4.5. Are We Acutely or Chronically Stressed?

4.5.1. The Situation Is Acute

If a stressor affects us briefly, our bodily stress reaction disappears as soon as the potential threat is over. In some cases, acute stress can cause an underlying illness to break out, for example, asthma or hypertension.

Potential triggers of acute stress are:

- permanent acoustic signals, for instance, alarms from medical devices
- time pressure
- lack of resources to accomplish the current task
- demands that are too complex
- acute tensions within a team
- ongoing interruptions
- mistakes which just happened
- unclear distribution of workload and responsibilities
- a sudden incidence which was not expected
- other triggers that you can name

4.5.2. Now, It Becomes Chronic

We speak of chronic stress when we are permanently under stress which does not cease.

Potential triggers of chronic stress are:

- too large a workload for too long
- an ongoing fight for lacking resources
- lacking support from supervisors

- too few personnel
- unpredictable rosters with changing shifts
- ongoing job-related confrontation with violence, injuries, and death
- competition and smouldering conflicts
- other triggers that you can name

This can compromise us mentally and physically. Potential consequences include illnesses such as hypertension, damage to the blood vessels with a subsequent heart attack, and even cancer.

4.6. How to Interpret the Signs Correctly

4.6.1. Signs of Acute Stress

Signs of acute stress are rapidly occurring reactions which are caused by our bodies´ transmitters. These are evolutionary age-old and prepare us to fight, escape, or to freeze. The transmitters, especially adrenaline, are disintegrated as soon as the stressful event is over.

Do you remember moments of shock, for example, a full braking because someone had ignored your right of way? We feel startled, react and relax as soon as the danger is over.

What we can feel:

- fright
- increased heart rate
- sweating
- faster breathing
- a decreased ability to think clearly

4.6.2. Signs of Chronic Stress

If we are under hyperstress or distress for too long a period of time with no relief in sight, this depressing situation will leave its mark.

Physical consequences include:

- sleep disturbance
- chronic pain and aches
- tense muscles
- stomach pain

Mental effects include:

- mood swings
- anxiety
- depression
- emotional burnout
- retreat
- irritability
- conflicts in relationships
- listlessness

Possible behavioural changes include:

- changed nutrition: too much, too little, or unhealthy food
- increased alcohol consumption and smoking
- consumption of illegal drugs or drug abuse
- imprudent and risky behaviour
- giving up physical training and other spare time activities

4.7. How to Manage Unwanted Stress Expertly

When examining unwanted stress, we are able to find the stressors and deal with them. In addition, we can take preventive measures. The earlier we do this, the better we can take care of our-selves and our capabilities, but we can also help stressed people around us. We find plenty of litera-ture on the following topics in books and online. Hence, let us consider them here as food for thought rather than studying them in-depth.

4.7.1. Why Do We Experience Stress?

First of all, it helps us to analyse which of the above mentioned types of stress we are experiencing and what the actual stressors are. Then, we should think about what further reasons for our stress exist. Are we lacking resources? Or do we feel that we are not capable of one or several of our tasks?

If so, we can take the next step and consider our opportunities, where and how to acquire the necessary knowledge and skills. Furthermore, we can think about our attitude, for instance, or about trust in our abilities and our expectations of ourselves.

4.7.2. How to Use Our Time

As described many times before, it is our task to allocate our time and to ponder what should receive our attention and what we need or want to leave out.

- What does really matter?
- What can we delegate?
- What can we rationalise?

Remember

In addition, we gain a lot of durable capacity if we reserve time in advance to relax, to meet dear people who are important to us, and to exercise.

4.7.3. When Exercising We Let Go of the Stress

Surely, you have experienced yourself how jogging in the woods or an exciting tennis match has helped you to relax and unwind.

Different sports effectuate the disintegration of different stress hormones, such as cortisol and adrenaline (2). Especially during endurance sports, endorphins are released. Last but not least, we are in a different environment, respond to a challenge, have fun, or enjoy being all by ourselves.

4.7.4. Nutrition and Stress

Top Quotation

"The best doctor is nature: She cures three quarters of illnesses and never speaks ill of her colleagues."

Louis Pasteur

Of course, we know which foods are healthy and rich in nutrients (fruit, vegetables, wholemeal bread, ...), but also, what we should stay away from, particularly when stressed. Everyone of us has his or her personal list. At this point, it is time for a huge praise to each of you, who is able to enjoy the items on your list in mod-eration.

Micronutrients, such as zinc, and iron, magnesium, and selenium carry out important functions in our bodies. We need more of them when we are in high demand. Scientists work eagerly to discover how these micro nutrients and stress mutually influence each other (3).

4.7.5. Sufficient and Restful Sleep

This topic keeps some of us awake at night as well. Ambitious people are kept on their toes until late at night by their workload, others brood over their worries. Some have been sitting in front of their com-puter screens too long yet again. Also those of us, who work at night or in shifts regularly, may have trouble falling asleep.

A lack of sleep and worrying about it may cause stress. At the same time, we are more likely to feel stressed when we do not sleep enough. As chronic sleeping disorders can impact our health, those affected should seek help.

Table 1 Types of Stress, Causes, Signs, What to Do

Types of Stress	Causes	Signs	What to Do
Eustress	an exciting challenge	we are focused, work hard	just keep going
Distress	a demand which exceeds our capacities; an incisive event in life, such as losing one's job, divorce	feeling helpless or hopeless; losing interest in one's activities, or friends; crying fits, bursts of anger; other physical, mental, or behavioural changes	depends on the situation, resources, and resilience; so, there is no easy general answer; counselling or even therapy might be necessary
Hyperstress	too many tasks, to few resources, lack of time, lack of instructions	difficulties to concentrate, to prioritise, to make decisions, or remember all tasks; physical symptoms include tense muscles, stomach pain, headaches and chest pain, amongst others	talk to supervisors/team members about how to share the workload, where to find resources, what to prioritise, etc.; exercise, adjust the diet, allow time for yourself, breathing exercises
Hypostress	too few tasks or tasks which do not match the knowledge and abilities	consequences include boredom, complacency, not feeling needed, substandard performance, not recognising one's scope of skills any more as it is narrowed	depending on the situation (temporarily, or not, etc.): talk to supervisors; new tasks or new definition of the role; if temporarily, use free time for further education
Acute Stress	acute occurrence, which startles us, acute stimuli	physiological signs of the flight or fight response, e.g., increased heart rate, faster breathing, sweating	acute stress will disappear as soon as the danger is over if caused by a single startling occurrence; otherwise try to stop the trigger
Chronic Stress	stress which goes on for a long time, too high a workload for too long, ongoing conflicts, too few personnel, unreliable rosters at work, etc.	mental, physical and behavioural changes; chronic diseases may develop, including hypertension, damage to blood vessels, leading to a heart attack, or cancer	identify the stressors; talk to supervisors/team members, be honest, try to find solutions which stop the stressors; if not helpful, a new job, or counselling might be needed; include exercising, nutrition, rest and sleep

4.8. Stress and Important CRM Components

If we bring personal stress to our teamwork, or a stressful situation arises at work, this will influence our crew resource management. Here, we will take a look at workload management, decision-making, and situational awareness as examples.

4.8.1. Workload Management

If we become distressed, we find it more difficult to prioritise our tasks correctly and to maintain an overview. Which tasks are important now, what is secondary? Who in our team should do what? Really relevant items can be overlooked and lead to a potentially major error in the process.

4.8.2. Decision-Making

When we are stressed and, on top of that, in a confusing situation, we may not be able to keep a cool head, which we need to make good decisions considering all the important aspects.

For instance, an ambulance crew may head for the wrong hospital, which does not provide the necessary department, because the crew has not considered all the possible differential diagnoses.

4.8.3. Situational Awareness

Our situational awareness is compromised when we are distressed. Consequently, an important piece of information from our environment may not reach us. For example, we may simply miss a team member's remark. In addition, we may notice dangers too late, as we have not paid attention to the warning signs earlier.

4.8.4. How CRM Helps Us in Stressful Situations

Here, we will take a look at standard operating procedures (SOPs) as well as checklists. Both are truly helpful tools in stressful situations.

Standard Operating Procedures

An SOP contains all the necessary steps of a procedure in the correct order or a flowchart. It helps us greatly not to forget anything if we have such a mnemonic in front of us, especially when we are distressed.

Checklists

Checklists contain all the relevant items, for example, all the equipment we need to secure a patient's airway in the emergency medical service. Using a checklist, we make sure that we have prepared everything and that we do not need to interrupt our procedure to look for utensils, which can be dangerous.

4.8.5. Addressing Challenging Situations in Training

Certain manoeuvres in aviation, such as landing an aircraft in extreme weather conditions, are naturally more stressful than standard situations. Therefore, they are rehearsed in simulators until the pilots master them confidently. If we are prepared to handle such a situation, we are used to it and, thus, become distressed less easily.

Top Tip

Congratulations, you have worked your way through a long chapter!

Now, what about enjoying a relaxed moment full of pleasure?

4.9. The Comprehensive Summary of Chapter 4

Concerning all types of harmful stress, their prevention and noticing signs early are crucial.

- eustress helps us to stay focused in the middle of a challenging task and reach our goal
- harmful types of stress include distress, hyperstress and hypostress, acute and chronic stress
- it is vital to know the definitions, the causes, and the signs of the different types of stress
- if we know definitions, causes, and signs, we can detect the respective type of stress early
- we should address the signs we have noticed and react personally and professionally
- we should take our time and allow ourselves to act preventively to build our resilience
- our CRM is impaired if we are stressed, but, in turn, CRM helps us to focus when stressed

4.10. More About Stress and CRM in the Next Chapter

We will deepen how stress influences important CRM components and elucidate the interplay of stress with these components. We will also reveal the role distress played in air disasters. Of course, we will turn our attention to training methods which prepare us to handle stressful situations.

4.11. References

1) Tan SY, Yip A (2018) Hans Seyle (1907-1982): Founder of the stress theory. Singapore Med J 59(4): 170-171. doi: https://doi.org/10.11622/smedj.2018043.

https://www.ncbi.nlm.nih.gov/pmc/articles/PMC5915631/pdf/SMJ-59-170.pdf, most recently accessed: July 23rd, 2023

2) Harvard Health Publishing, Harvard Medical School (2020) https://www.health.harvard.edu/ staying-healthy/exercising-to-relax, most recently accessed: July 23rd, 2023

3) Lopresti AL (2019) The Effects of Psychological and Environmental Stress on Micronutrient Concentrations in the Body: A Review of the Evidence. Adv Nutr 11: 103-112

https://doi.org/10.1093/advances/nmz082, https://www.ncbi.nlm.nih.gov/pmc/articles/PMC7442351/ pdf/nmz082.pdf, most recently accessed: July 23rd, 2023

5

5. Stress, Management and Relevance in CRM — Part II

These Contents Are Waiting for You in the Fifth Chapter

Stress of different causes can greatly influence the outcome of a flight. We will examine two examples of this, before turning our attention to various CRM components which help us to stay focused when stressed. Last but not least, how can we use CRM training to rehearse the appropriate handling of stressful events?

5.1. The Influence of Stress on Flights

Stress can either exist before the flight has even begun, or it is caused by an unexpected event during the flight. Both can lead to an incident or air accident.

5.1.1. Preexisting Stress Triggers an Incident

Stress, which pilots bring from their daily lives to their flights, becomes noticeable in their work. Although it is required by many sides or by ourselves as part of our professional conduct, we are not always able to separate our private lives and their influences on us from our occupation.

One incident, which luckily did not lead to an accident, shall be examined here. As the investigation of this incident showed, stress due to a financial loss in addition to disrupted sleep had impaired the captain's concentration (1).

When the pilot next to him, who was the pilot flying at this point in time, asked the captain to pull the landing gear up, the captain retracted the flaps on the wings instead. These flaps are used during take-off and climbing. At least, the captain had made sure that the airliner had already gained enough speed to carry out the manoeuvre securely. The crew noticed that the landing gear was still down at an altitude of 1000 feet (approx. 330m) and pulled it up.

5.1.2. Stressful Events Led to an Air Crash

On June 1st, 2009 an Air France Airbus , flight AF 447, crashed into the Atlantic Ocean en route from Rio de Janeiro to Paris (2). Only the discovery of the flight data recorder and the cockpit voice recorder in May 2011 revealed what had caused the accident, but also how the crew had acted during the last minutes of the flight.

Sensors, which measure the airspeed (pitot tubes), had frozen and, thus, the autopilot had disengaged. Consequently, the crew had to fly manually without reliable speed indication. In addition, a loss of altitude of about 160m was indicated, which had been wrong. This caused the pilot flying to pull the nose of the plane up making it climb.

He continued his manoeuvre until the airliner reached a point at which an aeroplane is not capable of flying any more due to aerodynamics. Instead, it begins to fall. The crew apparently misinterpreted the acoustic and visual warning sign and seemed not to believe that the aircraft was stalled. Thus, they did not return to a lower altitude in order to regain their speed, which would have recovered their aeroplane from the stall.

Following this, the crew concentrated on manoeuvres that did not yield the desired results, and their communication lost its mandatory discipline. Only right before the crash — much too late — one of the pilots recognised the cause, as well as the necessary action. Apparent stress (audible in the communication) caused by the events and further critical factors rendered the crew incapable of comprehending and solving the problem.

5.2. Stress Is an Important Topic in CRM

As you are well aware, stress influences our teamwork. The consequences can be fatal, as we have seen in the example above. This is the reason why the subject is taught so extensively in CRM.

Below, we will first address the interplay of stress and the CRM components. Using these components, we are still able to solve our tasks in a structured manner and to minimise mistakes when stressed.

Then, we will occupy ourselves with general CRM training and its goals. We will also look at targeted training of stressful situations in a simulation.

5.3. Stress and the CRM Components

5.3.1. The Interrelation Between Workload Management and Stress

Good workload management includes:

- clarity on the tasks
- clarity on who is capable of and going to do what
- overview of the tasks in relation to the situation as a whole
- overview in relation to time and progress, for example, during an entire flight
- overview of task execution
- timely and anticipatory planning of workload management, concerning time and personnel
- task fulfilment as soon as possible in order to have resources available in case of the unex-

pected

Using wise workload management we achieve i. a.:

- to avoid unnecessary stress due to uncertainty
- to avoid unnecessary stress due to inadequate preparation
- to avoid pitfalls employing adequate preparation, for instance, regarding the expected weather conditions during a flight
- due to anticipatory planning it is possible to prepare the appropriate actions concerning these conditions
- to detect lacking resources early, when there is still time to make amends
- to find potential faults in good time and to correct them early
- optimised professionality
- better teamwork

Adequate workload management is a relevant topic in CRM so that we master it even when we are feeling stressed.

Remember

If we maintain good workload management during stress, this helps us to keep an overview and continue our work calmly. Hence, we diminish the risk for mistakes.

5.3.2. Decision-Making

When applying CRM, we often decide as a team, and the team leader is responsible for the decision made. Especially when we are stressed, we tend to overlook important facts. Consequently, we find it more difficult to assess benefits and risks with certainty. Decision-making models serve us well particularly then. In the figure below, you can find examples of decision-making models and see, which aspects these include.

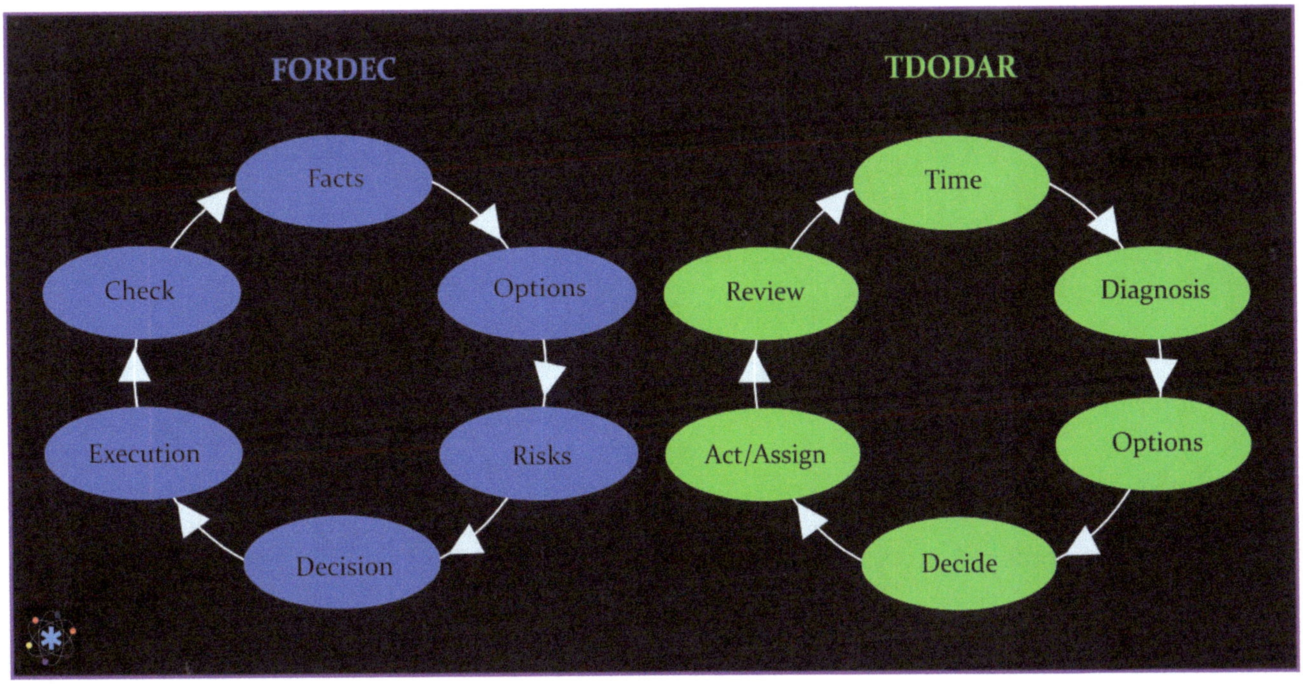

Figure 3 Examples of decision-making models, FORDEC and TDODAR

FORDEC, applied by well-known European airlines, as well as in medicine:

- Facts: What are the facts?
- Options: What options have we got?
- Risks: What risks exist?
- Decision: Who is going to carry out which task.
- Execution: Acting as decided.
- Check: Re-evaluation of the situation, adjustment of the measures if necessary.

TDODAR, applied by British Airways, for example, which has added "time":

- Time: How much time have we got?
- Diagnosis: What is the problem?
- Options: What options have we got?
- Decide: Who is going to do what.
- Act/Assign: Carrying out the tasks as decided.
- Review: Re-evaluation of the situation, adjustment of the measures if necessary.

5.3.3. Our Situational Awareness Deteriorates When We Are Stressed

When employing situational awareness, we comprehend our current situation as a whole. This includes:

- spatial awareness: when flying, but also in the emergency medical service in a labyrinth of a flat
- awareness of time: how far have we come in a procedure, how much time have we got left
- information from our surroundings, for instance, the weather during a flight, or crossing air traffic
- overview of the tasks or currently needed actions
- overview of the resources

Depending on the concentration that a situation requires, situational awareness can be divided into five levels, ranging from tuned out, for example, when lying on the beach, to comatose, caused by a startling event. We are most concentrated and, therefore, most alert when we are in the medium levels of awareness. The more tense we are, the shorter we can maintain a good situational awareness. When comatose, our situational awareness is limited due to the related stress.

Remember

A good cognition of our situational awareness, as well as the right mix of tension and relaxation also help us to deal with stress adequately.

5.3.4. Stress and Communication

When we are stressed, our ears can be "shut", remarks, but also warning signals, evade us. At the same time, our own communication can be incomplete. For instance, we may not stick to formal language, which is required in radio communication. We may speak fast and unarticulated or send misleading messages.

As you know, a lack in communication has lent a hand to about 70% of all air accidents. Therefore, the topic is truly important in CRM today. In addition, communication rules have been developed to enhance safety.

Remember

Closed communication loops, as well as the use of unambiguous standard phrases in CRM help us to continue to send and receive clear messages, even when we are feeling stressed.

5.4. CRM Offers Us Additional Valuable Tools

Standard operating procedures (SOPs) as well as checklists are of great help. Additionally, there are more mnemonics, as we will see below.

5.4.1. SOPs and Stress

We cannot apply safe crew resource management without following clearly formulated SOPs, neither in routine situations, nor in extraordinary ones that cause stress.

In many incidents and accidents in aviation deviation from the SOPs played a role (3). One example are the SOPs, which require a go-around in case of an unstabilised approach, in order to avoid a controlled flight into terrain (CFIT).

Factors, which contribute to deviation from SOPs, include:

- priority of other aspects such as maximal duty time
- overconfidence and complacency
- wanting to get the job done at all costs
- distractions
- interruptions
- stress and impaired situational awareness
- too large a workload
- lack of training in using SOPs
- lack of acceptance of SOPs in the company culture

Remember

In extraordinary and stressful situations, SOPs help us to solve the underlying problem step by step considering all important aspects.

SOPs for routine procedures help us to work stresslessly and flawlessly.

5.4.2. Relevance of Checklists During Stress

Imagine, you are doing the groceries, your mobile phone rings, a neighbour bumps into you and greets you. At the same time, someone wants to pass your shopping trolley and reach the shelf right behind you. Step by step you solve the situation, but what did you want to buy? Well prepared as you are, you grab your shopping list and get your shopping underway.

When we are at work, things are not that different. In the emergency medical service, we should not forget any item of our medical equipment when changing cars, but take all of it to the other vehicle. Such a change of vehicles can be necessary at short notice, for example, when a car is damaged. Of course, we should act quickly. As we cannot remember all items even when we are relaxed, this gets worse when we are feeling stressed. Then, we are glad to have our checklists.

Remember

Checklists help us to avoid stress caused by forgotten items and they help us not to forget anything when we are stressed.

5.4.3. Further Mnemonics

We are at a 78-year-old patient's place. One corner of his mouth is hanging down, his speech is slurred, perhaps he has suffered a stroke. His relatives are nervous, one tells us about a stroke three years ago, one provides us with the list of medications at the same time.

In order to continue to carry out or work calmly, remembering everything that is important, we use different acronyms in the emergency medical service. One of these is "FAST", shown below, which we employ when examining stroke patients:

- F for "face", is there any palsy?
- A for "arms", can one not be held up in front of the body?
- S for "speech", what are the pronunciation and the understanding like?
- T for "time", when did the symptoms first occur?

Remember

In addition to the items in the decision-making models, the SOPs and checklists, simple mnemonics help us to consider all the important facts when we are stressed.

5.5. General Training of CRM Components

As you already know, CRM comprises several components. Just reading them makes the mind boggle. Adhering to all these concepts in practical teamwork, requires a lot of practice through repeated training.

Remember

If we master the CRM components confidently, we will deploy them automatically and keep a cool head in stressful situations.

5.6. Specific Training of Simulated Stressful Situations

Imagine the Following Scenarios

An emergency landing after the outage of important onboard systems.

The rescue of an unconscious patient, this time trapped at the foot of narrow basement stairs, or high up in the driver's cab of a lorry.

How to deal with such stressful situations can be trained in a realistic simulation. In a simulator, no aeroplane can really crash, and no patient will be harmed. Moreover, the scenario can be repeated as often as necessary, until the team masters it successfully.

During the debriefing, the team members reflect together on what has been carried out successfully and what needs improvement. Peculiar attention is paid to the root cause of mistakes, which can then be addressed accordingly.

Top Tip

Simulation and the confidence we gain there minimise our stress level considerably when we are confronted with the practised scenario in reality. Thus, we reduce our risk of failure.

Considering that, we should use every opportunity to attend simulation exercises, despite our concerns about video recording and debriefing. Every instructor understands our fear.

5.7. Using CRM, Stress Can Be Handled More Easily

Having elucidated stress and its relevance in CRM, we have seen how the various CRM components and precise communication help us in stressful situations. Thus, it is easier for us to keep an overview and, as a team, to continue to use our personnel and material resources.

The continued training of the CRM components, as well as simulation with its detailed debriefing sessions, round off CRM uniquely. Equipped with it, we are better prepared to control our stress levels and fulfil our tasks with expertise.

5.8. The Comprehensive Summary of Chapter 5

CRM enables us to prevent unnecessary stress. CRM also helps us to continue when stressed.

- preexisting stress and stressful events on a flight can lead to incidents and air accidents
- stress is intertwined with CRM components and an important theme taught extensively

- good workload management helps to avoid stress and maintain the overview when stressed
- decision-making models help to consider all facts and provide structure
- a good cognition of situational awareness and knowledge of its five levels are important
- further aids to remember everything in complex situations: SOPs, checklists, mnemonics
- general CRM training as well as simulation training of stressful scenarios are beneficial

5.9. Next, We Will Explore an Extraordinary Emergency Landing

Following their brilliant start, the pilots on board a lordly Airbus A380 suddenly were confronted with a myriad of malfunctions. At first, they could not figure out why they had occurred and how they were interrelated. Although their airliner was severely crippled, they managed to land it without any casualties, an achievement that astonishes us to this day. We will highlight how the pilots used CRM to handle this event, which no-one had faced before.

5.10. References

1) Dr Graham & Daniel, Stress and Flight Crew, The Airline Pilots Forum & Resource,

https://www.theairlinepilots.com/forumarchive/aeromedical/stressandflightcrew.php, most recently accessed: July 25th, 2023

2) Final Report On the accident of 1st June 2009 to the Airbus A330-203, registered F-GZCP, operated by Air France, flight AF 447 Rio de Janeiro-Paris (July 2012), BEA, Bureau d'Enquêtes et d'Analyses pour la sécurité de l'aviation civile (Bureau of Enquiry and Analysis for Civil Aviation Safety)

3) https://www.skybrary.aero/articles/standard-operating-procedures-sops, most recently accessed: July 25th, 2023

6

6. CRM Travelling on an A380 to...

These Contents Are Waiting for You in the Sixth Chapter

Only minutes after take-off, two loud sounds on board Qantas flight 32 were followed by the loss of crucial flight controls. In addition to their superb knowledge, flying skills, and their professional attitude, the pilots used various CRM components to deal with the emergency and land the plane. We will also unveil, what other teams were involved and supported them.

6.1. The Departure After a Stopover in Singapore

6.1.1. Captain de Crespigny and His Crew

On the flightdeck of the mighty A380 were five pilots on November 4th 2010, which is unusual. Captain Richard de Crespigny, who was going to undergo a routine check, was assisted by his first officer Matt Hicks. Mark Johnson was going to be his second officer.

Also on board was check captain Harry Wubben, who was going to check captain de Crespigny, as well as one more check captain, David Evans. He was going to observe the checking pilot.

6.1.2. The Airliner

A Special Airbus A380 of the Renowned Airline Qantas

Qantas, the renowned Australian airline, which had its last deadly air accident in 1951, christened this A380 Nancy-Bird Walton after the legendary flight pioneer and placed it ceremonially into service in 2008.

Some Figures and Data

A lordly Airbus A380 is 72.73 metres long and has a wingspan of 79.80 metres. The maximum take-off weight is 560 tonnes. In this case, 105 of these were fuel. More than 500 passengers can be seated on board, the crew can comprise up to 35 persons. On Qantas flight 32, there were 440 passengers and 24 crew on board in addition to the five pilots. The four engines of an Airbus A380 can be delivered by two different manufacturers. In this case, they were from Rolls Royce, the Trent 900 model.

6.1.3. The Take-off of the Airbus A380

In Singapore, the weather was perfect for flying on this day in November, with sunshine and a mild wind. The first leg of the route had led here from London. After a stopover of two hours the new crew continued the flight to Sydney. Immediately before take-off, captain de Crespigny asked his crew: "Everyone happy?". His first officer Matt Hicks replied: "Yeah, just don't crash."

After an uneventful take-off from runway 20C at Changi Airport in Singapore, the aeroplane climbed into the sky without any difficulties heading South. Initially, it was flying over the Indonesian islands.

6.2. Two Loud Sounds on Board the A380

Only four minutes into the flight, at an altitude of 7000 feet, approx. 2330 metres, two loud sounds in short succession were heard in the cockpit of the A380. At this time, the airliner was flying over the Indone-sian island of Batam. Immediately thereafter, the aeroplane started vibrating. This is also visible on amateur videos taken by passengers (included in the informative film by ABC News, Australia, has been uploaded on YT) (1). At first, it was totally unclear what had caused the sounds. First of all, captain de Crespigny switched off the autopilot and abandoned the climb of the aircraft in order to level it.

6.3. Quickly, an Abundance of Occurrences Ensued

6.3.1. Malfunctions on Board the A380

The number-two engine, the inboard engine on the left-hand side of the plane, overheated. The message was conveyed to the crew via ECAM, short for electronic centralised aircraft monitoring. Right after that, ECAM started to show an abundance of further alarm messages on the respective display in quick succession. These referred to various onboard systems and, initially, there did not seem to be any connection between them. Then, ECAM reported that the number-two engine was on fire. Quickly, one after another, electronic and hydraulic aeroplane systems failed, amongst them the control over the brakes and slats, flaps and ailerons.

6.3.2. The Failures Caused Stress

The many acoustic and visual alarms, tied to the error messages, naturally caused stress, as did the at first apparently not interrelated events. Captain de Crespigny: "It was stressful, it was difficult." The crew had to cope with the stress in this very moment.

At the same time, every pilot involved knew that he had to apply everything he had ever learned about flying. Matt Hicks later said during an interview what he told himself after having briefly thought about his family at home: "Better do a decent job, otherwise I won't come home."

We will elucidate how the crew proceeded in correlation with the following CRM components and concepts:

- use of all resources available, concerning personnel, materials, inside and outside the A380
- workload management
- situational awareness
- decision-making
- knowledge, skills, and attitude
- appropriate communication
- threat and error management

Top Quotation Which Also Summarises the Quintessence of CRM

"I like to think that we sucked the brains´ drive, all the parts in the cockpit, to make one massive brain and then use the intelligence to resolve problems on the flight, because these were unexpected events, the unthinkable events."

Captain Richard de Crespigny, Qantas Flight 32

6.4. The Crew Applied Important CRM Components

First, it was vital to find the cause of the events, and to gain an overview of the situation as a whole, to stabilise the airliner, and to examine how the failed systems influenced the manoeuvrability of the plane. In addition, the crew had to plan further steps, and make decisions, inform the passengers, and prepare them for the emergency landing without causing panic on board. As you can see, there was a plethora of tasks, which the crew faced so suddenly and which it had to solve in order to bring all souls on board back to the ground safely.

6.4.1. Using Resources as a Team Immediately

The team in the cockpit used its members as resources and took advantage of the unusual presence of five pilots. The crew managed the workload wisely, as we will discover in subchapter 6.4.2. Thus, it was possible to gain an overview over the workload. At the same time, the workload was shared in a manner which allowed the crew to manage it.

Other teams were included as well, amongst them air traffic control (ATC) at Singapore Airport, the cabin crew, but also the passengers. It was crucial that they stayed calm. Contact with ATC in Singapore was made right away, and PAN PAN PAN was declared. This is the international sign that the aeroplane and its occupants are under threat, but the situation is not immediately perilous.

Secret

Help is a resource: What help will we be needing? Where can we obtain it? Help should be requested as soon as possible, and all persons involved should be informed as early as possible.

Furthermore, flying in a holding pattern was arranged with ATC for about thirty minutes in order to respond to the ECAM messages and to plan the rest of the flight.

Remember

It is vital to act anticipatorily: The holding pattern also served to keep the aircraft within gliding range, in case all onboard systems should fail.

6.4.2. Workload Management in the Cockpit of the A380

The Captain's and His First Officer's Tasks

Captain de Crespigny was going to fly the plane manually, which he declared formally using standard phraseology: "I have control."

First officer Matt Hicks took care of the ECAM messages. There were a total of 58 of them, which was unprecedented in aviation history. During training, responding to two or three of such messages in succession is practised.

Whilst Matt Hicks responded to the ECAM messages, he communicated relevant information to the crew and took action. For example, he shut down the number-two engine and later extinguished the fire using integrated mechanisms.

The Direct View of the Number-Two Engine

Second officer Mark Johnson took a direct look at the left wing from a window in the passenger cabin, as the wing cannot be seen from the cockpit. The wing was punctured. One of the holes was so large that a human being could have passed through it. The airliner was leaking fuel in sizeable quantities. The rear part of the nacelle was missing.

Back on the flightdeck, he communicated his observations to his fellow team members. It became clear that the engine had been destroyed, and that parts of it must have been blown apart cutting through various wires and hydraulic systems.

Calculating the Landing

The seasoned check captain David Evans calculated the length of the runway needed at the current weight of the plane, as it up until this point had barely used any fuel. Initially, the software indicated that a landing would be impossible.

After a discussion within the team and alteration of the parameters, there was a margin of 100 metres on a runway that is four kilometres long. The speed during the approach had to be controlled meticulously. If it had been too fast, the runway would have been overshooted, if had been too slow, the plane would have stalled and fallen out of the sky.

Collaboration with the Cabin Crew and the Passengers

In addition, David Evans informed the passengers in several announcements from the cockpit. Michael von Reth, the customer service manager, was involved right from the beginning as well. His role, as he attended to the passengers, was vital. He helped them to keep calm.

6.4.3. Decision-Making

After the initial sounds and the dramatic failure of the number-two engine, the impact of debris on the left wing, and the consecutive destruction of crucial aircraft systems, many decisions had to be made in order to land the aircraft on the safe ground.

Here are some of the decisions, the crew made in a short amount of time:

- to abandon the climb and level the plane
- to maintain a holding pattern for 30 minutes to respond to the ECAM warnings and to plan ahead

- to fly a left turn to see how the aircraft is responding
- who would perform which tasks
- to return to Singapore Airport requesting the longest runway
- requirement of the airport's fire brigade because of the fuel leak

In the meantime, parts of the A380 belonging to the engine and its nacelle, were found on the Indonesian island of Batam. On the nacelle, the airline's legendary kangaroo is visible. Indonesia's ATC informed the ATC in Singapore, which, in turn, passed the information on to the crew on Qantas flight 32.

Captain de Crespigny decided immediately that he could not deal with this message. At that moment, he was unable to do anything about it. Rather, together with his crew, he had to take care of the problems on board and the emergency landing.

6.4.4. Situational Awareness on the Flightdeck of the A380

As you know, situational awareness encompasses being conscious of the actual surroundings, and the time, as well as all accessible pieces of information, and the personal and material resources.

The crew was aware of the following information and resources and used them actively:

- **spatial:** distance to Singapore Airport, their altitude, distances and altitudes with respect to the emergency landing
- **time:** how much time do we allow ourselves to plan ahead, how much is too long and may cause problems
- **information:** what error messages are there, what is their cause, what has been destroyed, what does still work, the actual weight of the plane, weather conditions, including wind direction and speed
- **resources:** the pilots and their expertise, cabin crew, ATC and the possibilities at Singapore Airport, still available computer systems on board (e.g. landing calculation software), other systems that are still working

6.5. Knowledge, Skills, and Attitude

The knowledge, skills, and attitude of every team member are essential to the collaboration in order to use resources efficiently.

6.5.1. The Summarised Knowledge on Board the A380

Captain de Crespigny emphasised the value of the summarised knowledge on board as he said "…to make one massive brain and then use the intelligence to resolve problems…".

The knowledge on board comprised amongst others:

- general knowledge of flying
- general data and facts about the aeroplane
- the actual state of the A380
- where electric wires and hydraulic systems are located
- how the failures consecutively could be explained
- how to use the resources still available
- what runway and other resources on the ground were necessary for this kind of emergency landing
- where to find these resources, in this case the next major airport was Singapore

6.5.2. Flying Skills

In addition to the respective knowledge, practical skills were of enormous importance to handle the crippled plane and make the emergency landing successfully:

- flying a careful left turn to find out how the plane is responding
- performing a control check to explore the roll control right before the emergency landing
- using thrust wisely to control the speed precisely
- touching the stricken plane down expertly

6.5.3. Attitude Is Crucial, Too

The phenomenal teamwork attracts attention. We recognise that the available skills were combined at once: The knowledge was summoned into one massive brain and CRM was widely used.

6.6. Communication Inside and Outside the A380

Clear and explicit communication within the crew, as well as with other teams involved, was crucial for this success. We will first look at the various techniques used here. Then, we will reveal how many different parties communicated with one another in this case.

6.6.1. Communication Techniques

Speak up

The following examples can be named. Matt Hicks alerted the captain to the important speed regulation during the approach: "Watch your speed." Immediately after touchdown he requested several times that the captain brake maximally: "Brakes, Rich, Brakes."

Closed Communication Loops

Clearly stated and acknowledged were, for instance, the use of the integrated fire extinguisher in enginge number two, as well as the lowering of the landing gear before the emergency landing.

Standard Phraseology

As mentioned above, pilots clarify amongst themselves, who is flying the plane: Either stating "I have contol", or "You have control", which is acknowledged accordingly.

Sterile Cockpit Rule

During certain parts of a flight, especially during an emergency, the sterile cockpit rule applies. It says that all communication is now solely about the flight, the current situation and the tasks at hand. It is strictly forbidden to talk about private topics.

6.6.2. Who Communicated With Whom

When concentrating on the events on the flightdeck, one does not notice at first how many different parties were involved here and communicated with one another (Figure 4).

In detail, the following teams communicated with one another:

- the crew in the cockpit amongst themselves
- the cockpit crew with the cabin crew and the passengers

- the cockpit crew with the ATC at Singapore Airport
- Indonesia's ATC with the ATC in Singapore
- ATC in Singapore with the airport's fire brigade
- the Qantas operation centre, which monitors the whole fleet live, with ATC in Singapore (communicating with the cockpit was not possible due to the severed wiring)

All of that was important and had to be coordinated in order to make the emergency landing successfully and to support it, respectively.

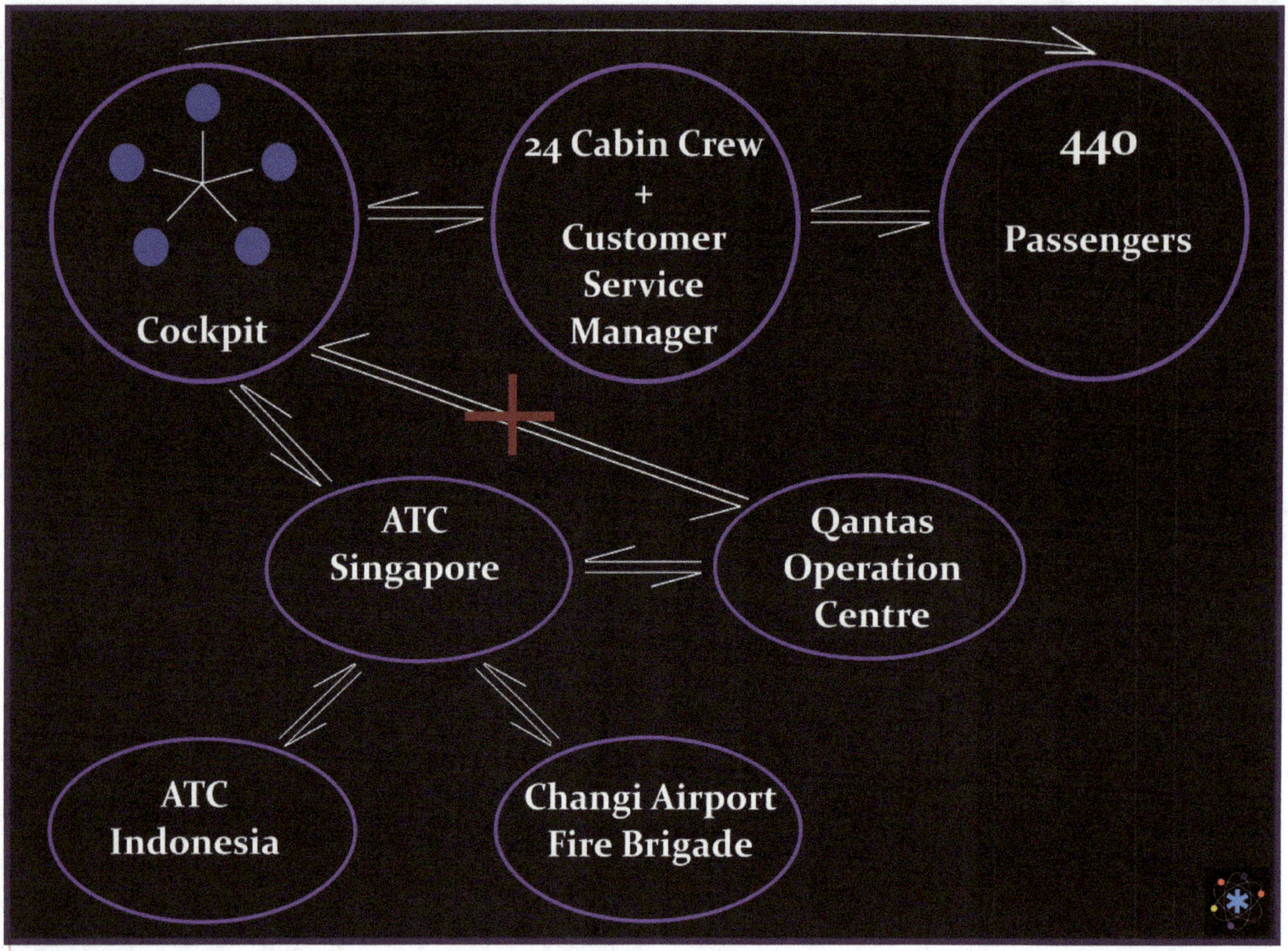

Figure 4 Qantas 32, communication between the parties involved

6.7. Threat and Error Management in the Cockpit of the A380

In crew resource management training, the avoidance, but also the management of threats and errors that have occurred nonetheless, is addressed in order to further enhance safety. A threat can also be caused by an error that has been made earlier and cannot be influenced by the crew.

On Qantas flight 32, the crew and everyone on board was severely threatened by the destroyed engine and the subsequent failures, without anyone having made an error during the flight. Now the crew had to deal with this already existing threat, which due to stress enhanced the risk of consecutive errors.

On the one hand, they achieved this due to preparation, including:

- consequent CRM training
- dealing with stress using CRM
- preparing for an engine failure and engine fire in a simulator
- practising an emergency landing and more in a simulator
- responding to ECAM messages during a simulation

On the other hand, not everything can be prepared. As mentioned above, it was the first time in aviation history that 58 ECAM messages were displayed one after another. It took fifty minutes in total to work through each one of them in order to be able to take the next step.

Also because of that, the management of the given situation was vital. This included:

- workload management
- dealing with stress right there and then
- gaining and processing information
- decision-making based on the information obtained
- communication
- employing the available knowledge, skills, and attitude, as well as all resources

6.8. The Emergency Landing in Singapore

6.8.1. Preparing the A380 for Landing

The hydraulic system of the landing gear was damaged as well. The crew lowered it manually and could only hope that gravity would pull it into place. This took a whole two minutes, but, luckily, it worked.

The cabin crew and the passengers had to be prepared for a hard and fast landing quickly. Everyone's collaboration in the cabin was essential.

Shortly before the landing, roll control was tested using a control check. It was severely limited, especially when the plane was rolled to the right.

The captain asked once more, whether nothing had been overlooked. After the acknowledgement, he started the final approach. Now he had to control the airspeed precisely down to a few knots (1 knot equals 1,852km/h).

6.8.2. The Actual Landing

After touching down on the runway, de Crespigny pushed the nose down as quickly as possible in order to avoid that tyres would explode when braking due to lacking contact with the ground. Such an explosion is only a question of split seconds.

Due to the failure of the braking system, only manual braking was possible. Matt Hicks reminded the captain several times to brake hard, because the plane did not seem to slow down. The latter replied that he was braking maximally already, which could be confirmed by looking down onto the brake pedal.

Captain de Crespigny saw the fire brigade as it was standing by, he aimed at them: "They were my friends." The huge A380 came to a halt one hundred metres within the end of the runway right next to the fire engines.

6.8.3. The Danger Was Not Over Yet

Already in this moment, the crew and the passengers were incredibly happy. However, the danger was far from over after this superb emergency landing. Fuel was leaking from the left wing in large quantities, the temperature of the brakes directly under it was exceeding 900 degrees Celsius. It goes without saying what consequences this could have had.

Using a coded message directed to the cabin crew, everything was prepared for an emergency evacuation. During such an evacuation, everyone on board has to leave the aircraft within ninety seconds.

The number-one engine, the outboard engine on the left-hand side, could only be shut down after several hours. For this, fire extinguishing foam was applied.

Only after two hours, the passengers could be evacuated from the right-hand side of the plane. Their relief was boundless. As one passenger later recalled: "I was thinking of kissing the ground."

Remember

In the chaos of this first-time event in aviation, well structured CRM, efficient communication, as well as knowledge, skills, and attitude aided the crew to manage their stress levels and to master the emergency landing.

6.9. Are the A380 and Its Engines Safe? - The Investigation

6.9.1. Assessing the Damage Directly After the Landing

Having left the airliner, the pilots took a look at the engine. They were shocked by the view. The rear part of the nacelle was missing, the aft section of the engine was held in place solely by the turboshaft. The traces of the fire were visible, as was the damage to the wing and its joint to the fuselage.

6.9.2. Inspection of the A380 Parts in Indonesia

Immediately after the engine parts had been found on the island of Batam, specialists of the Australian Transport Safety Bureau (ATSB) were dispatched to start the investigation there. Luckily, no one on the ground had been hit by the falling debris.

One part of the turbine disc, which weighs more than two hundred kilogrammes in total, was found in the detritus. A blue tinge on it suggested that a leaking lubricant might have caused the engine explosion.

The discovery of the parts confirmed a so-called uncontained engine rotor failure (UERF) i. e. a destruction during which debris flew out of the engine, hit the wing and its joint to the fuselage, severing the control systems. Luckily, the upper section of the fuselage was not hit by the part of the turbine disc that had punctured the wing. The fuselage is not constructed to withstand such an impact.

6.9.3. Examination of the Engine in Singapore

The airliner was towed to hangar 6. There, the engine was dismantled until the technicians could see the spot where the fire had started.

An untight oil pipe was discovered from which a lubricant had leaked onto hot parts of the engine and, subsequently, had caught fire. Consecutively, parts of the turbine structure had overheated, the turbine disc had started to spin at uncontrollable speed and, finally, had exploded.

6.9.4. The Root Cause of the Leakage

The cause of the leakage was a stub pipe which was sitting in a borehole which had not been drilled in a straight fashion. Besides, the wall of the stub pipe was too thin (2). Due to the strain during take-offs on short runways, cracks had formed in that stub pipe over time. On flight 32, the pipe became totally untight.

Remember

The faulty stub pipe represented the error, which developed into a threat to the crew and all the passengers during the flight.

6.9.5. Consequences for the Refitting and Maintenance of the Rolls Royce Engines

The stub pipe, which is only five centimetres long, had not been suitable for the engine. Therefore, all the engines of the same kind have been refitted accordingly. Besides, Rolls Royce has taken measures to prevent uncontained engine failures. The company has improved its quality management system as well.

Remember

Even **after this incidence, the painstaking investigation of the cause has** helped to avoid another event of this kind. Thus, it has made flying even safer.

6.10. The Comprehensive Summary of Chapter 6

Superb teamwork with CRM and a professional attitude helped the pilots on Qantas flight 32 to withstand the stress and apply their vast knowledge and skills expertly.

- after an uncontained engine failure, multiple system failures ensued rapidly
- an unprecedented number of 58 ECAM messages appeared, alarm bells sounded
- the pilots did not panic, but used their resources to handle an event never seen before
- they took advantage of the enlarged crew in the cockpit and distributed the workload wisely
- they quickly involved other crews and communicated sufficiently, also to the passengers
- the pilots used their situational awareness, made decisions, and dealt with the threat
- working closely together, also during approach and landing, they saved all souls on board

6.11. Threats? Errors? Don't Panic, We Will Explore Next What to Do

Above, we have already taken a brief look at how to manage threats and errors successfully. We will explore this topic further in the next chapter. In addition, we will elucidate what an undesired aircraft state (UAS) is. How does it happen? What are the consequences? What learning points can we transfer to our own lines of business?

6.12. References

1) ABC News Australia (2011, presented anew 2020) Four Corners, VIDEO: QF32: Retracing the story of the Qantas A380 mid-air explosion, https://www.abc.net.au/news/2020-11-03/qf32/12844570, most recently accessed: July 26th, 2023

2) Australian Transport Safety Bureau (2013) ATSB Transport Safety Report Aviation Occurrence Investigation - AO-2010-089, Final. In-flight uncontained engine failure overhead Batam Island, Indonesia, 4 November 2010, VH-OQA, Airbus A380-842

7

7. How to Keep Threats and Errors in Check Skilfully

These Contents Are Waiting for You in the Seventh Chapter

Threats can cause errors, and errors can become threats. What have they got to do with an undesired aircraft state? Looking at one item at a time and using practical examples, we will elaborate all the necessary definitions and untangle the interrelations. Of course, we will highlight the value of various CRM principles which help us to manage threats and errors expertly.

7.1. Examples, the Beginning, and Interrelations

7.1.1. Threats and Errors in Our Daily Lives

We are driving in our car on a country road, the sun is about to set, and right in front of us a sounder of wild boars runs onto the road. We brake immediately and manage not to hit this sounder.

This was a threat from the outside, without anyone having made a mistake. We could not help it and dealt with the situation deftly.

Still lost in our thoughts, we go on. Suddenly, our good friend in the passenger seat shouts: "Brake, for god's sake, you have to give way, and someone is coming!" We brake hard, the lady who has the right of way does the same. At the last second, a collision is prevented.

Due to the threat before, which had still compromised our concentration, we almost made the mistake not to give way.

For the driver on the main road we were a threat as we speeded towards the crossroads. Both of us reacted, the mistake was corrected in time. Thus, it had no consequences other than the amazement.

Additionally remarkable here is our good friend's speak up. He had noticed the danger and alerted us immediately (Figure 5). The speak up is an important element in the communication used in crew resource management. It helps us as a team to recognise errors in good time.

Remember

Threats come from the outside. We can predict some of them and prepare ourselves. Others are unpredictable. Threats require action and render a situation complex.

Errors, however, occur when someone has done something wrong, be it in the communication, during a procedure, or when driving a vehicle.

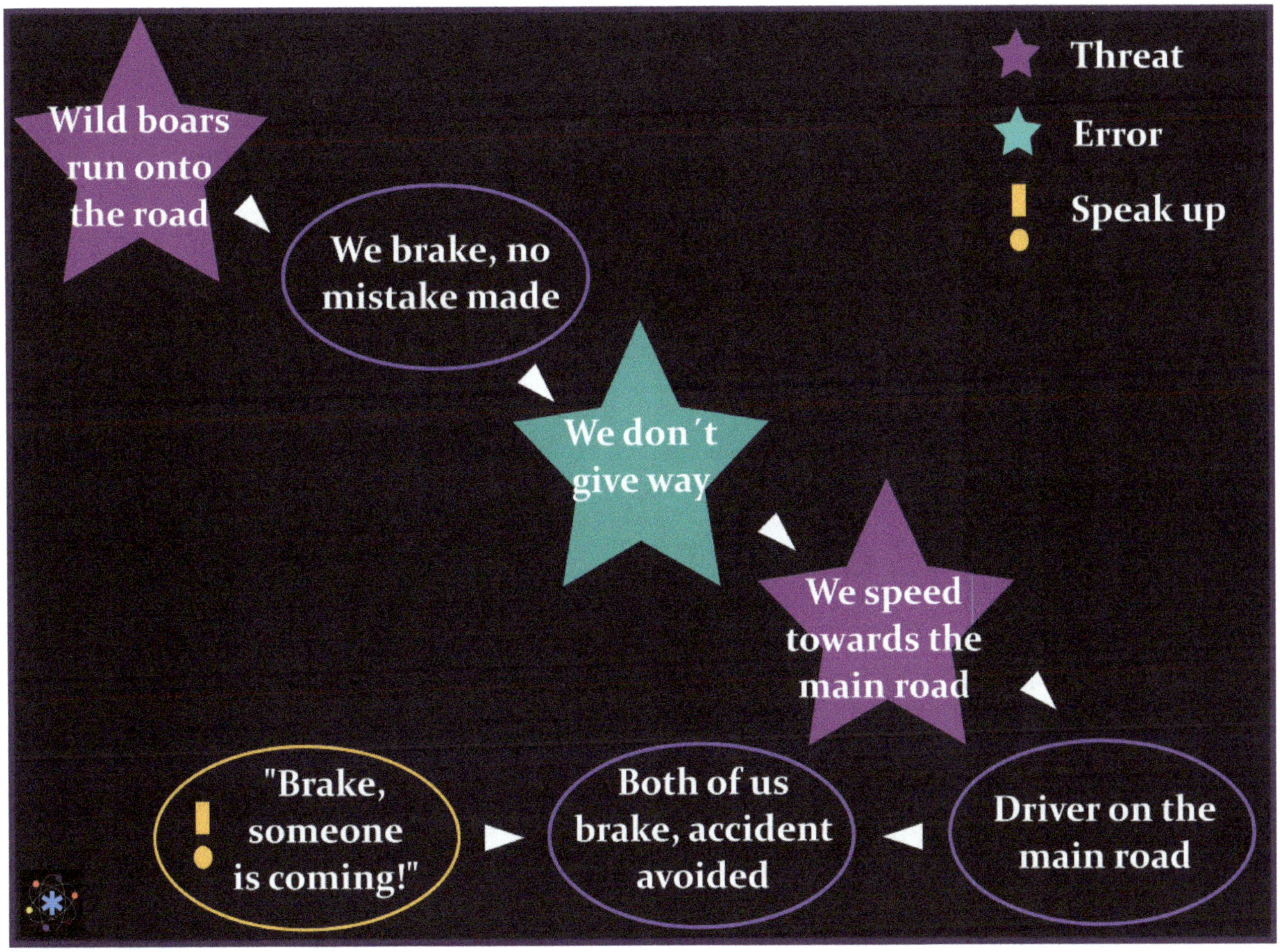

Figure 5: Example of threats, an error, and a speak up

7.1.2. The Awareness of Threats and Errors Is Established

The beginning dates back to 1994, when the University of Texas and Delta Airlines initialised a joint project. During so-called Line Operation Safety Audits (LOSA) pilots are checked during routine flights. The focus is on what threats occur during a flight and how the crew responds to them. In addition, it is on errors and undesired aircraft states. Today, LOSA is fully established. It is not about avoiding threats and errors altogether, since that is not possible. It is about how to minimise them in advance and/or how to deal with them before threats and errors cause real harm.

7.1.3. Connections Concerning Threats and Errors

Errors Lead to Threats and Vice Versa

Threats distract us from our duties, we have to react to them first. Our situational awareness suffers. Sometimes, we even startle upon the threat, our concentration and our ability to think clearly are compromised. Hence, mistakes can easily happen.

On the other hand, a threat can be the result of an error. For instance, when preparing for a medical procedure, important material may be forgotten. Naturally, the utensils are needed exactly when the situation becomes complicated, a hectic rush ensues, the flow is disturbed, subsequent faults become all the more likely.

Errors, Threats and Human Factors

The human factors such as "lack of concentration", "lack of knowledge", and "lack of assertiveness" (taken from the so-called "Dirty Dozen"), as well as insufficient communication, influence our successful management of threats and existing errors.

At the same time, errors occur due to the human factors, which we will examine in subchapter 7.5.

How to Avoid and Deal with Threats and Errors Successfully Using CRM

Threat and Error Management (TEM) (1), dealing with threats and errors is taught as an important topic in Crew Resource Management. As we will elucidate in subchapter 7.6., CRM components that are used otherwise as well, help us to avoid and successfully manage errors and threats.

7.2. Threats in Aviation

7.2.1. Threats Have Different Causes

In every phase of a flight, a wealth of threats can happen. Some are not confined to a single phase of a flight. Examples include:

On the Ground

- insufficient signage
- closed or contaminated taxiways or runways

During Take-off

- ATC instructions that are difficult to follow
- language difficulties
- mistakes on the part of ATC

In the Air

- all imaginable technical malfunctions and failures on the aeroplane
- delays and resulting time pressure

During Landing

- weather conditions such as strong winds, or thunderstorms
- a wet or icy runway

7.2.2. Two Threats Combined

The Crash of a Small Passenger Aircraft

On 8 January 2003, a Raytheon (Beechcraft) 1900D, Flight Air Midwest 5481, with 21 souls on board, plunged from the sky onto the premises of Charlotte-Douglas International Airport in North Carolina, USA, immediately after take-off.

Sadly, no one on board survived the disaster. Captain Katie Leslie managed at the last moment to avoid hitting a hangar with many people and aircraft inside, which saved many others´ lives.

The Air Crash Investigation

The excellent investigation by Lorenda Ward and her team from the National Transportation Safety Board (NTSB) revealed the cause of the crash (2). Two independent threats had combined in a fatal manner, as we will discover in a moment. There were no pilot errors.

This air crash investigation is retraced in the truly recommendable film „Mayday 05 – Dead Weight" , it contains interviews, amongst others (3). The film is available on YT as well.

Maintenance Errors on the Elevator

Due to errors during maintenance, the elevator was not fully deployable. Thus, during too steep a climb, the nose of the plane could not be lowered. The steep climb was caused by too heavy a weight aft.

Wrong Standards Were Used when Calculating the Overall Weight

The heavy weight due to too heavy baggage on board was not an error in the pilots′ calculations. It resulted from decades old, far too low assumptions for the average weight of passengers and baggage. According to the standards, the pilots had not used the actual weight of all pieces of luggage and passengers in their calculations.

Remember

The painstaking investigation of air disasters helps to make aviation continuously safer. Also in this field, threat and error management is applied.

7.3. Errors in Aviation

7.3.1. Definition of Errors in Aviation

Errors in aviation are actions or inactions of the crew which

- lead to a deviation from the intentions or expectations of the crew or the organisation
- reduce safety margins
- can lead to adverse events

7.3.2. Sources and Examples for Errors in Aviation

Errors in aviation concern aircraft handling, procedures, and communication. Examples include:

Errors with Respect to Aircraft Handling

- wrong speed or altitude
- wrong thrust, wrong position of the flaps
- wrong runway or taxiway

Procedural Errors

- missing important items during briefing
- disregarding standard operating procedures or government regulations
- flawed documentation

Errors in the Communication

- with ATC
- the crew in the cockpit amongst themselves
- with the cabin crew

7.3.3. Reporting Errors for Continuous Improvement

Just as threats, crews report errors to the reporting system of the airlines.

Remember

These error reports, their processing, and the drawn conclusions are an important part of TEM.

7.4. Undesired Aircraft State (UAS)

On our road trip we speeded much too fast towards the crossroads. Our car was in an undesired state so to speak, which we had caused by our mistake. There was no technical failure of the brakes.

Remember

Thus, the undesired state results from an error and not from a threat. It reduces the safety margins.

The same applies to aircraft. As opposed to threats, for instance, the engine fire on Qantas flight 32 (chapter 6), the undesired state is due to errors the crew has made.

Examples of undesired aircraft states include:

- taxiing the airliner onto the wrong runway
- wrong altitudes in any phase of a flight

- wrong heading
- insufficient line-up with the runway on the approach

It does not take much imagination to work out the consequences of an UAS. Collisions can happen on the ground, in the air, but also with the surrounding terrain, called controlled flight into terrain (CFIT). Hence, it is important that the pilots prioritise to correct the error and eliminate the UAS as soon as they notice it.

7.5. Errors, Threats, and Us - How to Master Human Factors

We all know how it feels to be too tired, or to have far too little time, where we lack the necessary knowledge despite all our efforts, and where we have miscommunicated. These human factors (4) are sometimes presented as the "Dirty Dozen" along with other definitions:

- fatigue
- stress
- pressure, real or self-induced
- distraction
- complacency
- lack of resources
- lack of communication
- lack of teamwork
- lack of assertiveness (speak up)
- lack of knowledge
- lack of attentiveness
- norms (attitude and habits)

Remember

If we look at this Dirty Dozen during CRM training and apply appropriate solutions, we minimise its potential influence and, thus, our risk of errors.

7.6. Threat and Error Management is Part of CRM

7.6.1. The Philosophy of Threat and Error Management (TEM)

The philosophy of TEM emphasises three essential concepts: anticipation, recognition, and recovery.

Anticipation

Generally speaking, we anticipate that threats and errors cannot be avoided, but will certainly appear. However, it is not clear, where and when. Therefore, we maintain the vigilance which is important in all safety-critical professions.

This vigilance helps us to recognise threats and errors.

Recognition

As soon as we recognise errors and threats, we can act and induce countermeasures. This leads to:

Recovery

As we attend to the error or threat, we recover the safety margins in the first place. Depending on our line of business, we make sure that errors or threats do not influence a patient's safety, the safety of a flight, or other procedures.

Remember

It is imperative to recover first and analyse the causes later.

7.6.2. How the Particular CRM Components Help Us

Using different examples, we will elucidate the important and valuable role that CRM components play in the recognition and the handling of threats and errors.

Situational Awareness

If we maintain our situational awareness concerning space and time, available information, as well as personal and material resources at any time, we are able to detect threats early and to use our resources to react properly.

Examples:

- spatial: dense air traffic around the airport, threats caused by other airliners, collision avoidance necessary
- time: a patient's compromised circulation after an accident, rapid measures and transport are necessary
- information: There are heavy thunderstorms at the destination as a threat, should one aim for another airport?

Communication

Matter-of-fact, clearly formulated messages, which are confirmed, help us to point out the relevant items unmistakably and to make sure that the message is understood.

Using a 10-for-10, the 10-for-10-concept means ten seconds for the next ten minutes, we discuss as a team, using a scheme, what problems exist, what steps are necessary in the next minutes, and how we are going to distribute the workload. When there are no more questions, we start working as agreed.

Managing Stress

As stress impairs our ability to think clearly and to act, we need to keep our stress in check (chapters 4 and 5). As in an interrelationship, the CRM components help us with that. Of great help are also deliberate relaxation, a positive attitude, as well as the confidence in our well-trained skills, which we bring to our teamwork.

Workload Management

If we know the personal resources in our team well, we are able to distribute the workload wisely when facing a threat. In the emergency medical service, the increasing swelling of a patient's airway is a threat. We have to recognise this early and decide, whether an intubation in general anaesthesia, as well as ventilation, are needed. If so, we discuss briefly, who is going to prepare what and who is going to perform what tasks during the procedure.

Gaining and Processing Information

Gaining information early and actively is advantageous in order to recognise threats quickly.

Decision-Making

We observe the situation, gather information, also regarding threats and errors. Using our resources, such as team members and auxiliaries, we decide how we are going to proceed.

7.7. Threats and Errors Successfully Minimised

If we are aware of the presence of threats and errors, their different types and underlying human factors, we are able to counter them using our resources.

7.7.1. We Master Anticipatable Threats

During simulator training sessions, probable threats are anticipated and the appropriate responses are rehearsed. Such threats may be engine failures during a flight, or rescuing people from a vehicle that is about to burst into flames. If the situation occurs, we startle less easily, we do not freeze in shock. We handle the procedure more confidently with an optimised result. Hence, the risk of ensuing errors is reduced as well.

7.7.2. More Capacities to Deal with Unexpected Threats

If we apply CRM consistently, we are aware of the possibility that unexpected threats may occur at any time. If we are vigilant a priori, if we work as a team in a well-structured manner and finish our tasks swiftly, we have more capacities for the unexpected.

7.7.3. We Make Anticipatable Errors Less Often

If we rehearse and discuss potential causes of errors consequently, we recognise the errors we are able to avoid in the first place. Examples include the confusion of different medications. As we look at the ampullae together whilst we prepare the syringes, we can keep the risk of a mix-up at bay.

7.7.4. Minimising the Consequences of Errors

Starting with appropriate communication (speak up, closed communication loops), moving on to the use of mnemonics (have we really prepared everything?), and ending with the continuous re-evaluation of our steps and measures as a team, we try to spot possible errors immediately, before they have any consequences.

Before the departure in the ambulance to a hospital, we check whether the entire monitoring, including heart rate, blood pressure and oxygen saturation, is established. We also check whether we have prepared every medication we might need en route, but also whether we have informed the right hospital in advance. If we find any omissions now, we can still correct them.

7.7.5. We Grow as We Investigate Threats and Errors

Secret

Whenever we have encountered threats, or made an error, we discuss these constructively. What did we do well, where is still room for improvement? What can we learn for our next calls?

7.8. Master Threats and Errors in Your Line of Business

Now you have read intently for a long time, which is a huge achievement! If the topic is new to you, of course, you cannot remember everything at once and apply it right away.

Are You Ready?

After revision (if necessary), don't you fancy a challenge and wish to put your new knowledge into action step by step? Imagine going ahead together with your team and celebrating your resulting successes.

Anticipate, Recognise, Recover

What threats and errors do you anticipate in your profession? How can you recognise them? What will you do to recover?

The Vexatious Human Factors

What human factors play a role in your line of business? What steps can you take in your work environment?

Using CRM Components

Where can you use CRM in order to minimise errors and threats?

7.9. The Comprehensive Summary of Chapter 7

Recognising threats and errors early and understanding how they are intertwined with the human factors and CRM helps us to minimise their impact.

- a threat comes from the outside, it can be the result of an error and prompt the team, which faces the threat, to make an error
- an error is the result of a wrong action or communication, it reduces the safety margin and can develop into a threat
- an undesired aircraft state (UAS) is due to an error, e.g. wrong altitude or heading
- some threats are predictable, others occur unexpectedly, they make a situation complex
- threats and errors cannot be avoided altogether, thus, TEM teaches us how to deal with them
- the philosophy behind TEM is: anticipate, recognise, recover, act first, analyse the cause later
- we need to be aware of the human factors which may cause us to make mistakes
- helpful CRM components to be used in TEM include: situational awareness, communication techniques, managing stress,workload management, gathering and processing information, decision-making
- after having encountered a threat or having made an error, we should always analyse them to learn from them and take measures to avoid the respective mistake in the future

7.10. Our Next Topic Will Be the Error Chain

Unfortunately, it is not as beautiful as a string of pearls: the error chain. It originated in aviation, too. How many links has it got? How many of these are necessary to cause an air accident? How can we prevent fatal errors using this knowledge?

7.11. References

1) Merrit A, Klinect J (2006) Defensive Flying for Pilots: An Introduction to Threat and Error Management. The University of Texas Human Factors Research Project. The LOSA Cooperative. https://skybrary.aero/sites/default/files/bookshelf/1982.pdf, most recently accessed: July 27th, 2023

2) National Transportation Safety Board, NTSB (2004) Aircraft Accident Report, Loss of Pitch Control During Takeoff, Air Midwest Flight 5481, Raytheon (Beechcraft) 1900D, N233YV, Charlotte, North Carolina, January 8, 2003, https://reports.aviation-safety.net/2003/20030108-0_B190_N233YV.pdf, most recently accessed: July 27th, 2023

3) Mayday - S05E05 - Dead Weight (Air Midwest Flight 5481), https://www.dailymotion.com/video/x8l6kbz, most recently accessed July 27th, 2023

4) 1) https://skybrary.aero/articles/human-factors-dirty-dozen, most recently accessed: July 31st, 2023

8

8. The Error Chain and How to Disrupt It Successfully

These Contents Are Waiting for You in the Eighth Chapter

Below, we will distinguish the error chain from a chain of events before examining each of its eleven links separately. As we go along, we will look at various examples and the respective definition before we unveil which of the CRM principles help us to break each link. We will round this chapter off with three real cases from routine medical work, each of which represents one link of the error chain.

8.1. The Examination of Air Accidents Led to the Error Chain

When a group of researchers analysed more than 300 incidents and accidents in aviation, they discovered that only rarely one single human mistake had preceded these events. In addition, only seldom had one member of the team been responsible. Mostly, several team members had made errors.

The researchers looked at the errors in the light of the human factors and, consequently, developed the model of the error chain with its eleven links (1). Each of the links represents a kind of behaviour or an experience, which can lead to mistakes, as we will discover in subchapter 8.3.

8.2. What We Need to Know About the Links of the Error Chain

8.2.1. Important Figures

On average, seven of the eleven links were present in the more than 300 examined air accidents and incidents. The minimum, which was detected in the events, was four links of the error chain. Generally speaking, the risk of an incident or accident rises if links of the error chain surface during a flight.

8.2.2. What Can We Deduct From the Figures for Ourselves?

Pause and Think

Does that mean that an air accident will be prevented if the pilots let only happen three of the links during a flight?

If we transfer the concept to our work, will we always be on the safe side if we allow a maximum of three links to occur in one piece of work?

Of course, there is no one hundred percent guarantee, as potentially momentous events depend on the nature of the combined links and additional factors. However, we minimise our risk for grievous errors considerably.

8.2.3. The Error Chain Seen Before and After an Event

In hindsight, especially as a spectator watching from the outside, one is always smarter than everyone who had acted during the actual event. Hence, it is also easier to verify the links of the error chain during the investigation of an air accident. Will this simple insight bar us from occupying ourselves with the error chain preventively?

Remember

If we know the meaning of the links, we can recognise them in our work actively.

If we address them using the appropriate CRM concepts, we can break them.

8.3. We Look at the Eleven Links Separately

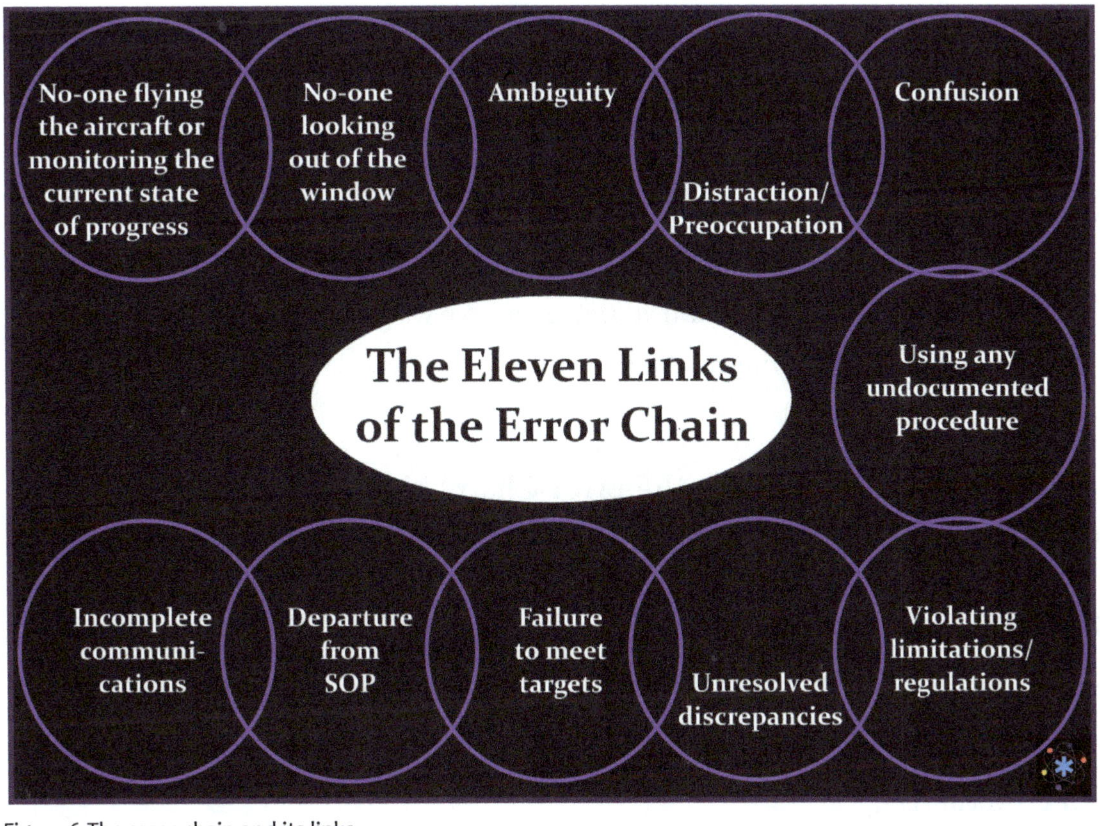

Figure 6 The error chain and its links

In the figure above, you can find the meaning of the links. We will take a look at them one at a time, using examples from our everyday lives (as appropriate) and a description. Furthermore, we will highlight which CRM concepts we can apply in order to break the error chain.

8.3.1. No-One Flying the Aircraft or Monitoring the Current State of Progress

An Example From Everyday Life:

Imagine, you are preparing a meal together with others. The pasta is already being boiled. A question about an ingredient for the sauce suddenly attracts all attention. In the meantime, the pot with the pasta overboils with a whiz. Everyone was occupied with a single ingredient, whilst no-one was cooking.

Description:

The pilot flying (PF) flies the plane, whilst the pilot monitoring (PM) monitors the systems and the progress of the flight in accordance with the actions of the PF.

In situations in which both take their attention from these duties and tend to one problem only, no-one is flying the aircraft any more. Thus, threats and errors (chapter 7) might be detected and dealt with too late.

CRM concepts which may help:

- situational awareness: spatially, as well as concerning time, information, and resources, we keep an eye on the situation as a whole
- workload management: What duties/problems have we got? Who will do what?
- decision-making: What priorities have we got to set in what order?

8.3.2. A Self-Explanatory Link of the Error Chain: No-One Looking out of the Window

Description:

If none of the pilots is looking out of the window, a mid-air collision can happen, especially in areas with heavy air traffic.

A helpful CRM concept:

Situational Awareness, in this case spatial awareness.

8.3.3. Ambiguity

Example:

You are invited to a cool party by two people. However, each of them tells you a different date. As you absolutely must attend this party, naturally, you do not rest until you have found out the correct date.

Description:

During a flight, the pilots may obtain different specifications from various instruments, crew members, or air traffic control. Now, they have to find out which piece of information is correct.

Helpful CRM concepts:

- communication: clarification through double-checking and reconciling of specifications
- speak up when someone has noticed a discrepancy in order to call on the team to sort the situation out
- 10-for-10-concept: in ten seconds the team plans the steps it will take during the next ten minutes

8.3.4. Distraction/Preoccupation

Description:

Distraction in aviation can be due to bad weather, technical malfunctions, or a high workload, but also private problems. The crew may be involved in a problem, which has occurred all of a sudden, so deeply that it fails to recognise additional threats or mistakes early.

CRM concepts you can use:

- situational awareness
- communication in order to discuss the circumstances and the measures to be taken
- workload management
- wise use of all resources

8.3.5. Confusion as a Link of the Error Chain

Description:

Uncertainty, anxiety, or bafflement can be possible triggers of confusion. This holds particularly true if pilots reach the boundaries of their knowledge or their skills, notably if the situation is new to them. Consequently, mistakes tend to happen more easily.

CRM concepts which bring clarity:

- workload management in order to keep an overview of the situation
- good teamwork which creates an atmosphere in which uncertainties are discussed openly
- communication: for example, briefings regarding possible problems on the flight

8.3.6. Using Any Undocumented Procedure

Description:

Checklists, manuals, or standard operating procedures (SOPs) cannot be written for every imaginable situation in advance. Hence, a crew has to deal with events which have not been documented yet. In this case, it is important to clarify whether the crew understands the current problems and the potential consequences.

An important difference to link number ten of the error chain is the nonexistence of written documents, whereas they, logically, in the case of a deliberate deviation do exist.

CRM concepts which should be applied first:

- using all available resources as a team: Have they really all been applied to their full potential?
- 10-for-10-concept in order to discuss all options together
- decision-making, also employing standardised models, for instance, FORDEC or TDODAR (chapter 5.3.2.)

8.3.7. Violating Limitations/Regulations

Example:

Someone has left far too late for a previously arranged lunch with a relative. Now, alone on the rural road, this person flouts the speed limit and drives a bit too fast. If we also have done this ourselves before, we must admit that it was deliberately in these cases.

Description:

As in the example above, this is about the intention to potentially violate a limitation or to actually overstepping it. In aviation, limitations pertain to a wide variety of items such as rest periods, maximum number of working hours, but also airspeed limits.

Possible CRM concepts:

- communication: assertive speak up of a team member
- knowledge, skills, and attitude: here, it is about professional attitude, but also about the knowledge of the limitations (chapter 3)

8.3.8. Unresolved Discrepancies are Part of the Error Chain

Description:

As in our daily lives, discrepancies in aviation can relate to opinions, information, but also changing conditions.

CRM concepts:

- good teamwork from all members in order to address discrepancies constructively
- communication: addressing discrepancies assertively and suggesting solutions
- shared mental model: ensuring that everyone has got the same picture of the situation

8.3.9. The Failure to Meet Targets Belongs to the Error Chain

Description:

In aviation, the failure to meet targets includes, for instance, the estimated arrival time (ETA), an assigned level or heading.

When a crew fails to meet a target, this is not considered done deliberately. Thus, it is not a violation of regulations as in subchapter 8.3.7.

Helpful CRM concepts:

- workload management in order to keep an overview, to recognise tasks and then assign them to persons, as well as time slots
- wise use of all personal and material resources
- timely communication of the goals, discussion of the progress

8.3.10. Departure from SOPs

Description:

Here, a crew deviates from existing SOPs. Organisations write SOPs as solutions to potentially problematic situations. Pressure, complexity, and a lack of time may precede such deviations.

CRM concepts:

- using all available resources as a team, before such a departure from an SOP becomes necessary
- applying the 10-for-10-concept in order to discuss all options together
- decision-making including the use of standardised models

8.3.11. Incomplete Communication

Example:

You have not been given important instructions concerning a task and now you are wondering how to proceed. Due to the incomplete instructions, you have to spend time and make an effort to obtain the information you need.

Description:

On the one hand, incomplete communication means withholding important information, opinions, suggestions, and questions. On the other hand, we also subsume miscommunication here, during which discrepancies are not resolved.

CRM concepts:

- communication techniques: closed loop communication, standard phraseology, speak up
- knowledge, skills, attitude: showing a professional attitude, we convey all the information we have
- good teamwork: a working atmosphere in which we can sort ambiguities out

8.4. The Error Chain Is Not a Chain of Events

As we have seen above, the eleven links of the error chain are clearly defined and pertain to the human factors. Thus, they highlight human errors which are made before an accident.

A chain of events, however, contains environmental factors, as well, such as adverse weather conditions or technical malfunctions. These, in turn, can trigger the links of the error chain: For instance, a technical problem may attract everyone's attention, whilst no-one is flying the aircraft any more.

8.5. We Recognise and Break the Links in Our Work

Pause and Think

When you look at the error chain and its links, which of them surface in your profession or daily work? Which CRM concepts would you use to break them?

Let us now look at a few examples from the medical world, which have happened in reality.

8.5.1.No-One Is Resuscitating the Patient

During simulator training, but, unfortunately, also in real emergency rooms it has occurred that everyone involved participated in securing the patient's airway. Thus, no-one carried out the all-important chest compressions for several minutes.

8.5.2. Confusion in the Emergency Department

A young doctor with only little experience has to stich a wound on the head of a small, crying child in an overcrowded emergency department. Right before she starts, her consultant reprimands her harshly in front of the parents and the child due to the treatment she had offered another patient.

You can easily imagine that in this situation her startling, the child who cannot be calmed down, her inexperience, and the pressure created by the never-ending stream of patients confuse the young doctor. How can she now produce a fine suture with non-shaking hands?

8.5.3. Unresolved Discrepancies on the Scene

On an emergency scene, the ambulance crew meets a middle-aged patient with chest pain, a cough and dyspnoea. The ECG shows abnormalities. The team fails to communicate their tentative diagnosis clearly amongst themselves. Following that, two team members think of a myocardial in-farction, the other two of a pulmonary embolism. Hence, the team has no shared mental model, rendering their joint treatment difficult.

8.5.4. Constructive Debriefings Including the Error Chain

As you certainly are aware, in these three cases solely constructive debriefings are helpful, during which the experts involved elucidate, which links of the chain were present and what they will do differently next time.

Pause and Think

Is such a debriefing possible in every working atmosphere?

We can only work on this together.

8.6. The Comprehensive Summary of Chapter 8

The error chain represents human factors with its eleven links and must not be confused with a chain of events.

- after examining more than 300 incidents and air accidents, the error chain was established
- each link represents one human factor, either a behaviour or an experience
- on average, 7 links were detected, the minimum was 4 links in each case
- keeping the number of links below 3, minimises the risk of a momentous mistake
- however, there is no guarantee, as the combination of links and other factors play a role, too
- we should know the links and the helpful CRM concepts in order to break them
- it is beneficial to use the error chain in hindsight to prevent the reoccurrence of detected links

8.7. Next, We Will Apply the Error Chain

Using the worst air accident, which has happend so far, as an example, we will shed light on what circumstances and factors belonged to the chain of events and where we can detect links of the error chain. In addition, we will discover that not only one person made an error.

8.8. Reference

1) https://navyflightmanuals.tpub.com/P-1283/Identifying-Links-In-An-Error-Chain-41.htm, most recently accessed: July 30th, 2023

9

9. The Chain of Events on the Island of Tenerife

These Contents Are Waiting for You in the Nineth Chapter

When two jumbo jets collided on the island of Tenerife in 1977, a chain of many circumstances, technical failures, and human factors contributed to this accident. It was the worst one in civil aviation so far and took the lives of 583 people. We will discover what links of the error chain played a role in addition to the fatal chain of events. Furthermore, we will explore what changes have been made following the air crash investigation in order to enhance the safety substantially. This outlook is crucial when we deal with such a dolorous topic.

9.1. A Chain of Dramatic Circumstances

9.1.1. An Explosion on the Island of Gran Canaria

On Sunday, 27 March 1977, a bomb exploded at the airport of Gran Canaria. Police closed the airport and searched it for further explosive devices. Large airliners, among them two Boeing 747s were diverted to the airport Los Rodeos on the island of Tenerife.

A KLM jumbo jet, flight number 4805, came from Amsterdam. The other one with the flight number 1736 belonged to Pan Am and was on its way from Los Angeles to the Canary Islands after a stopover in New York.

The explosion and the following diversion of the flights are the first two links in our chain of events.

9.1.2. We Find More Links of the Chain of Events at Los Rodeos Airport

Los Rodeos is a small airport located 632 metres above sea level. As it lies at the foot of the mighty volcano Pico del Teide, it is often coated in fog which descends from the mountain. At this airport, which normally only handles small, regional aeroplanes, there was no ground radar at that point in time. In addition, the runway centreline lighting was out of service.

In the tower, there were only two air traffic controllers on duty as was the norm on Sundays. They were not used to heavy air traffic, not to mention jumbo jets. The flight crews of the aircraft arriving on this day were instructed to park on the taxiway, because the air traffic controllers had no other choice.

Between the taxiway and the runway there are four access lanes, C1 to C4. Number 1 and 2 were not accessible any more due to the aircraft which were sitting on the tarmac. Number 3 and 4 are shown on the accident sketch in the ICAO Circular 153-AN/56 on page 57 (1).

9.2. The Catenation Continued

9.2.1. A Wait of Hours

The KLM airliner was sitting in front of the Pan Am jet at the edge of the taxiway. The crew from the Netherlands (Captain Jacob Veldhuyzen van Zanten, First Officer Klaas Meurs, flight engineer Willem Schreuder) decided to take on 55 tonnes of fuel here already in order to save time in Gran Canaria. After all, they still had their return flight to Amsterdam ahead of them. The crew was concerned that they might exceed their maximum time of duty.

The Pan Am crew (Captain Victor Grubbs, First Officer Robert Bragg, flight engineer George Warns) descended from the cockpit to find out whether they would be able to get past the KLM airliner and onto the runway. However, 3.7 metres of space were lacking, which is little considering the wingspan of 59.6 metres of both planes.

9.2.2. Heading Towards the Take-off Position in Thick Fog

By the time the possibility to fly on to Gran Canaria finally had arrived, Los Rodeos Airport was shrouded in thick fog. With visibility ranges partially below 300 metres, the aircraft were sent to the end of the runway one after another. To reach this position, they taxied along the runway and not along the taxiway, because of the planes which were parked there.

The pilots were instructed to follow one another directly. There was no waiting until an aircraft had taken off safely. The KLM team was to perform a 180 degree turn in order to position their airliner for take-off. The Pan Am team was to use exit C3, which branches off the runway at an acute angle.

9.2.3. Captain van Zanten Released His Brakes, the Pan Am Team Was Looking for Exit C3

Captain van Zanten was ready for take-off, his first officer told air traffic control: "We are now at take-off". The sentence might have also been "We are now — uh — takin′ off." This could not be distinguished clearly by listening to the existing recordings. In the first case, the airliner would have been in its take-off position, in the latter, it would have been in the process of taking off. The air traffic controller seemed to be puzzled as well. He replied: "O.K. (pause), stand by for take-off, I will call you." The pilots of the Pan Am jet, whilst they were looking for exit C3, answered immediately via radio that they were still on the runway. ATC asked them to report runway clear as soon as they would have left it.

ATC never issued take-off clearance to the KLM crew. Nonetheless, van Zanten released his brakes and started to accelerate the massive aircraft as his first officer was still communicating with ATC. Willem Schreuder, the flight engineer, however, heard the radio message of the Pan Am crew and dared to speak up. He asks Captain van Zanten whether the Pan Am might not have left the runway yet. The captain replied emphatically: "Oh yeah!" Having been rejected in this manner, the flight engineer did not dare to insist.

9.3. Collision on the Runway

The Pan Am copilot was the first to see the KLM jumbo jet as it emerged from the fog. Upon his yelled "get off, get off, get off", captain Grubbs turned left sharply and opened the throttles fully at the same time. In the cabin, the passengers and personnel were shaken heavily.

At that moment, van Zanten realised that the Pan Am airliner was right in front of him on the runway. He yanked the control column towards himself so sharply that during that attempt to take off the tail section of the KLM aeroplane scratched the runway. The front wheels could be lifted over the top of the Pan Am, but not the outer engine on the right, which stroke the fuselage of the Pan Am. Also due to the 55 tonnes of extra fuel, the airliner was too heavy for that.

Subsequently, the KLM jet hit the runway and burst into flames immediately. The Pan Am airliner caught fire as well. In addition, its engines were still running and started throwing pieces of metal around. 61 passengers and nine crew members of the Pan Am plane managed to escape the burning wreckage. Unfortunately, nine of these passengers succumbed to their injuries later.

9.4. The Investigation Identified Technical and Human Failure

Experts from Spain and the Netherlands carried out the aircrash investigation.

9.4.1. A Heterodyne Destroyed Vital Parts of Radio Messages

The examination of the cockpit voice recorder showed that there had been a heterodyne when ATC had been talking to the KLM team whilst the first officer of the Pan Am crew had been announcing simultaneously that they were still taxiing down the runway. Hence, the KLM team could only understand the "O.K." of the sentence "O.K., stand by for take-off, I will call you", whereas the rest of the sentence became inaudible due to a garbled noise.

9.4.2. The Missed Exit as Another Link in the Chain of Events

The wreckage of the Pan Am jumbo jet was found between the exits C3 and C4, which clearly leads to the conclusion that the crew had missed their exit. The reasons for this additional link in the chain of events may have been the thick fog and distraction due to the radio message of the KLM crew, as well as the fact that the team was not familiar with the airport layout. Furthermore, the access lanes were not clearly marked.

9.4.3. Possible Training Syndrome

Captain van Zanten had last worked as a trainer in the simulator most of the time. There, the concentration lies exclusively on the flying manoeuvre which is being practised. Therefore, his situational aware-ness during the real flight, in which all pieces of information from the surroundings must be taken into account, may have been compromised.

9.4.4. The Exit C3 at an Acute Angle May Have Been Inaccessible for Jumbo Jets

Exit C3 branches off the runway at an acute angle. As experts stated after the investigation, it might be almost impossible for pilots of jumbo jets to make a turn at that angle. As the air traffic controllers had no experience with such large aircraft, they may not have thought about that.

Taken together, we can see that a chain of circumstances, which had partially already existed before the landings at Los Rodeos Airport, technical failures and human factors contributed to the disaster. You can find them summarised in the figure on the next page.

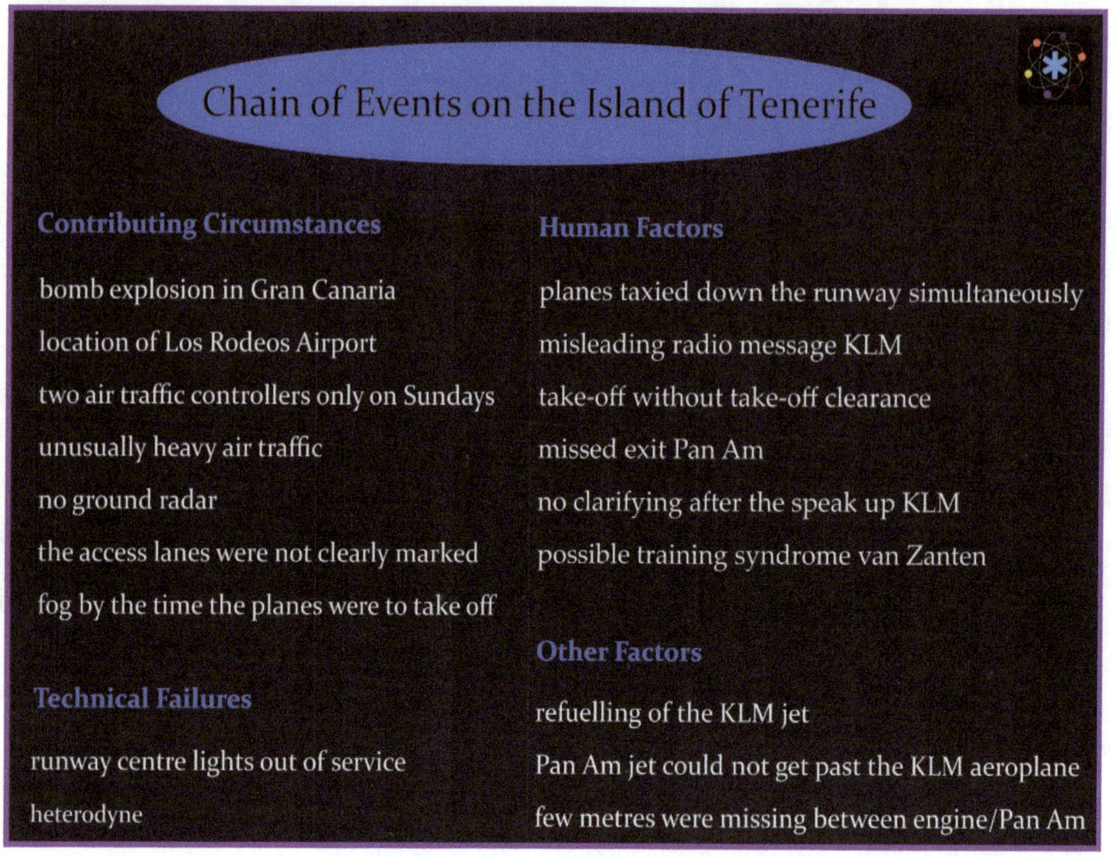

Figure 7: The Chain of Events on the Island of Tenerife

9.5. A Short Repetition of the Error Chain

As explained in chapter 8, the examination of more than 300 incidents and accidents in aviation has led to the error chain with its eleven links (2). In this model, the eleven links of the error chain are clearly defined and refer to human factors.

A chain of events, however, as we have seen above, contains also other factors, such as the fog and the heterodyne in this example. Now, after a short repetition of the error chain, using the figure provided again below, we will explore, which of the links we can detect in this chain of events.

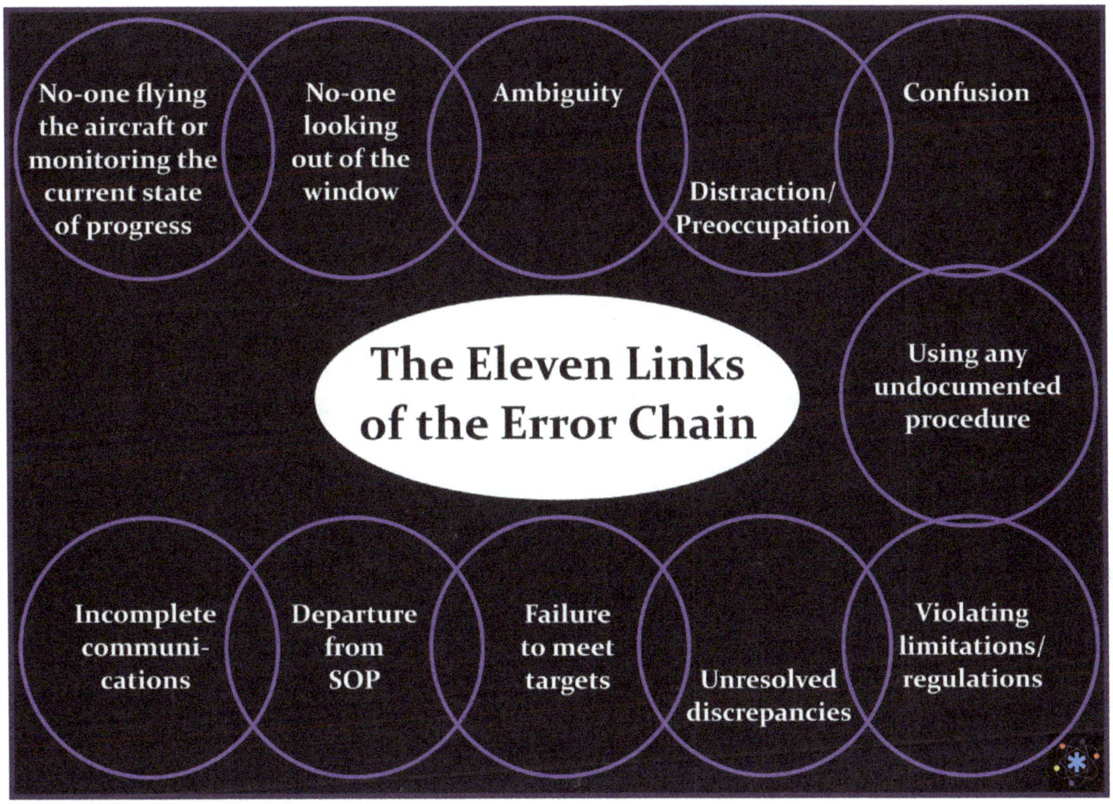

Figure 6: The error chain and its links

9.6. Finding the Links of the Error Chain in the Chain of Events

Pause and Think

Look at the chain of events in subchapter 9.4. again. Which of the links of the error chain can you recognise?

9.6.1. Distraction/Preoccupation

The Pan Am crew was distracted by the radio message of the KLM team whilst taxiing down the runway. This is one of the reasons why they missed their exit.

Due to their concerns about exceeding their maximum time of duty, the concentration of the KLM crew may have been compromised.

9.6.2. There is Much Confusion in This Chain of Events

We can only try to put ourselves in the position of the teams which were in the middle of these events. The initial situation alone with so many aircraft at Los Rodeos and the bomb explosion, the long wait and the uncertainty about when and how things would progress, has certainly contributed to the confusion.

Air Traffic Control

The two air traffic controllers had to coordinate too many flights at a time and too large planes without ground radar in thick fog in an unusual situation.

The misleading radio message of the KLM copilot: "We are now at take-off/we are now - uh - takin' off" certainly created another moment of confusion.

The Pan Am Team

The Pan Am team was confused by radio message from the KLM crew as well. The copilot reacted immediately. As we can see here, distraction can add to the confusion.

We can only try to imagine, what the passengers and cabin crew experienced in terms of confusion during the entire event.

9.6.3. Using Any Undocumented Procedure

As this is an unprecedented event, much of what happened at the airport refers to this link of the error chain:

- aircraft were parked on the taxiway
- the pilots were told to use the runway to taxi into position
- both the jumbo jets taxied almost directly one after another to their take-off position
- one jumbo jet was required to make a turn at an acute angle

9.6.4. Unresolved Discrepancies

After the flight engineer's speak up no clarifying took place.

9.6.5. Failure to Meet Targets in Various Links of the Chain of Events

- the KLM team ran the risk of exceeding its maximum time on duty
- on the whole, all the deviated flights were delayed for hours
- the Pan Am crew missed exit C3

In all these cases, no deliberation can be detected. Thus, there was no violation of existing rules on purpose.

9.6.6. Incomplete Communication

The sentence "We are now at take-off"/"we are now — uh — takin´ off" was misleading (ICAO Circular 153-AN/56, page 62 and following).

Due to the heterodyne, an important part of the answer was lost.

The speak up did not lead to a re-evaluation of the situation. If a team does not resolve a discrepancy using appropriate communication, the communication remains incomplete here as well.

9.6.7. Violating Limitations/Regulations

A violation of limitations/regulations can be discussed concerning the take-off without take-off clearance. However, this take-off was also caused by non-standardised phraseology and the heterodyne, which is why we should be cautious with our interpretation.

9.7. Conclusion Chain of Events/Error Chain and What No-one Had Expected

We can recognise some of the links of the error chain easily. Partially, it is not possible to clarify in hindsight, what was really going on within the teams. Nevertheless, we are able to detect more than three links of the error chain in the accident.

On the basis of the links of the error chain identified, we can see that several members of the respective teams required or carried out actions which contributed to the crash. These are intertwined with the chain of events.

That no-one had reckoned with the following, certainly contributed to these actions:

- ATC may not have expected that the Pan Am crew missed the exit
- the Pan Am team had certainly not expected the sudden take-off of the KLM jet
- ATC had not expected that take-off without take-off clearance either
- all three teams had not expected the heterodyne and the loss of information

9.8. Resulting Improvements of Safety in Aviation

During the lengthy and meticulous air crash investigation, light was shed on all its facets. From these, various institutions and authorities derived measures to maximise aviation safety.

Overview of the measures taken:

- a new airport on the island of Tenerife at sea level
- ground radar at Los Rodeos Airport
- standardised communication on the radio
- first generation of CRM: flattened hierarchies in the cockpit and speak up
- a blocking device for airliners to prevent heterodynes, not mandatory yet

In remembrance of the 583 victims,

but also of those who were severely injured

and mentally traumatised.

9.9. The Comprehensive Summary of Chapter 9

A complex chain of events, consisting of external and technical factors, interrelated with human factors, represented by the links of the error chain, led to the worst civilian air accident so far.

- the air traffic controllers at Los Rodeos airport faced a situation which they were not trained

to manage, namely suddenly taking care of many aircraft, including two jumbo jets
- other links of the chain of events included: no ground radar, thick fog, the airport layout
- the air traffic controllers sent the aircraft directly one after the other along the runway
- Pan Am crew (not familiar with the airport) had to take an exit lane at an acute angle
- misleading statement by the KLM crew, not clear whether they were already taking off
- ATC never issued take-off clearance to the KLM crew
- important links in the chain of events: missed exit, possible training syndrome, heterodyne
- very important, also with respect to today's CRM: the speak up KLM's flight eningeer made, however, at that time, he did not dare to insist
- the links of the error chain: distraction/preoccupation, confusion, using any undocumented procedure, unresolved discrepancies, failure to meet targets, incomplete communication, violating limitations/regulations (the last one should be discussed with caution)
- improvements include: a new airport on Tenerife Island and ground radar at Los Rodeos, standardised communication on the radio, first generation of CRM, flattened hierarchies
- the device on aircraft, which prevents heterodynes, still not mandatory yet

9.10. What is Just Culture?

The example showed us impressively that the speak up was not followed by an according reaction. Furthermore, it was not repeated assertively in the culture which prevailed at that time. What has changed since then? Moreover, what do we mean by "just culture" in CRM?

9.11. References

1) ICAO Circular 153-AN/56, which contains:

1. Title page: Raad voor de Luchtvaart, Netherlands Aviation Safety Board, Final Report and Comments of The Netherlands Aviation Safety Board of the investigation into the accident with the collision of KLM flight 4805, Boeing 747-206B, PH-BUF, and Pan American flight 1736, Boeing 737-121, N736PA, at the Tenerife Airport, Spain, on 27 March 1977.

2. The Spanish Report (October 1978) Part 1 (The Investigation, page 22 = first page, and following) and Part 2 (Analysis and Conclusions, page 42 and following).

3. Comments of the State of Registry (Kingdom of the Netherlands), page 57 and following.

The ICAO Circular can be downloaded from: https://www.faasafety.gov/files/gslac/courses/content/232/1081/finaldutchreport.pdf, most recently accessed: July 23rd, 2023

Links to the Spanish Report in English Part 1 and 2:

http://www.project-tenerife.com/engels/PDF/Spanish_report.PDF, most recently accessed: July 29th, 2023

http://www.project-tenerife.com/engels/PDF/spanish_report2.PDF, most recently accessed: July 29th, 2023

2) https://navyflightmanuals.tpub.com/P-1283/Identifying-Links-In-An-Error-Chain-41.htm, most recently accessed: July 30th, 2023

10

10. Just Culture

These Contents Are Waiting for You in the Tenth Chapter

How do we feel when mistakes almost automatically lead to punishment without any possibility to clarify what the circumstances were like? What are the consequences of such an approach? In contrast, what would be the results of a work environment without any sanctions at all? Everyone of us is well aware that we need a sensible way to deal with unintentionally made mistakes, but also gross negligence. This is where just culture comes into play. Below, we will explore its development and main features before we will elucidate how to create it at our own workplaces.

10.1. How Just Culture Was Established in Aviation

1.1. A Punitive or Blaming Culture

Mistakes Were Not Supposed to Happen

As in many industries and businesses, in aviation mistakes were not expected to occur. If someone had made an error nonetheless, he or she was held accountable, regardless of whether he or she really was to blame. Had there been any circumstances contributing to the mistake? What risks had existed already? Who else had been involved? These important questions were not asked. Rather, the focus was on the search for a scapegoat and disciplinary measures.

Hidden Mistakes

As we know from our own lives, such a management of mistakes leads to a demoralising atmosphere in which fear of punishment prevails. Consequently, we feel that it is at least very tough to admit mistakes and take responsibility for them. Every now and then, someone will try to hide an error completely.

Missed Learning Opportunities

In addition, the organisation as a whole cannot obtain important insights into the causes of errors, crucial learning opportunities for everyone are missed. Hence, what is to be seen as a positive chance to eradicate an error permanently and, subsequently, to enhance safety, is lost.

Something Crucial Was Missing

The culture of avoiding mistakes at any cost was usually accompanied by a power gradient. In this overall atmosphere, there was no place for a speak up, which plays an important role in today's crew resource management.

As a consequence, warnings about potential risks and further questions if someone was about to make an error were non-existent. Moreover, how should one have dared to pass on important information after having been rejected several times before? This also held true in healthcare for a long time, when a resident presumed to question the instructions given by a consultant constructively.

10.1.2. A Non-Punitive or No-Blaming Culture

Trend Reversal in the 1990s

In aviation, it was noticed that due to the hiding of mistakes vital information, which was much needed in order to improve safety, was lost. Furthermore, one tried to mend the damage, which had been caused by constant fear and pressure. Now, employees were encouraged to report mistakes and risks, as well as to contribute to safety concepts. Improvements of aviation safety were achieved.

The Atmosphere Should Not Be too Relaxed

As the reporting of mistakes involved amnesty, these were now being reported, but the organisation was seen as accountable for them. The employees expected not to be punished. This went so far that dangerous behaviour was even shown deliberately and repeatedly, which enhanced the risk of an unfavourable outcome. After all, one was not held accountable. It goes without saying that these were the boundaries of the concept.

10.1.3. Just Culture Was Created From These Insights

As we have seen, the above mentioned oppositional approaches were not ideal. Using these insights, just culture was created, which we will discuss below.

10.2. This Is Just Culture

10.2.1. Justice Is Important When Dealing With Mistakes

Just culture stands for justice when assessing and punishing mistakes or searching for their root causes. Was the mistake made by a single person or is there a flaw in the system? What measures are therefore necessary? Was the mistake made inadvertently or deliberately? By the way, he term "just culture" has never been translated into German. Therefore, the concept is known as "just culture" in German aviation as well.

10.2.2. The Characteristics of Just Culture

Below, you will find the fundamental criteria of a just culture at a glance:

- a culture without any unfounded blame or punishment
- anyone can make a mistake at any time, regardless their position
- everyone has clearly defined tasks and responsibilities
- mistakes and potential risks should be reported honestly
- a speak up is valued
- errors are assessed justly, causes are explored
- the root causes are eliminated as far as possible, risks are minimised
- after anonymisation of the mistake, a learning opportunity for everyone is created
- if guilty, the people involved are held accountable according to the previously agreed conditions
- gross negligence will be punished according to the regulations of the respective line of business, up to the loss of a professional licence

10.3. Professionalism Is Vital

Remember

A just culture to deal with mistakes and risks does not mean that an overall reduced performance is allowed.

Everyone has to know his or her tasks and how to accomplish them with the right knowledge, skills and appropriate attitude. Moreover, everyone has to be aware of his or her responsibilities.

Especially high performers with huge expectations of themselves feel extremely uncomfortable when making mistakes. All they can do afterwards is to take the bull by the horns, admit the error, apologise and review it constructively together with their team, if applicable. The role, which just culture plays in the correction of errors, is also depicted in Figure 8.

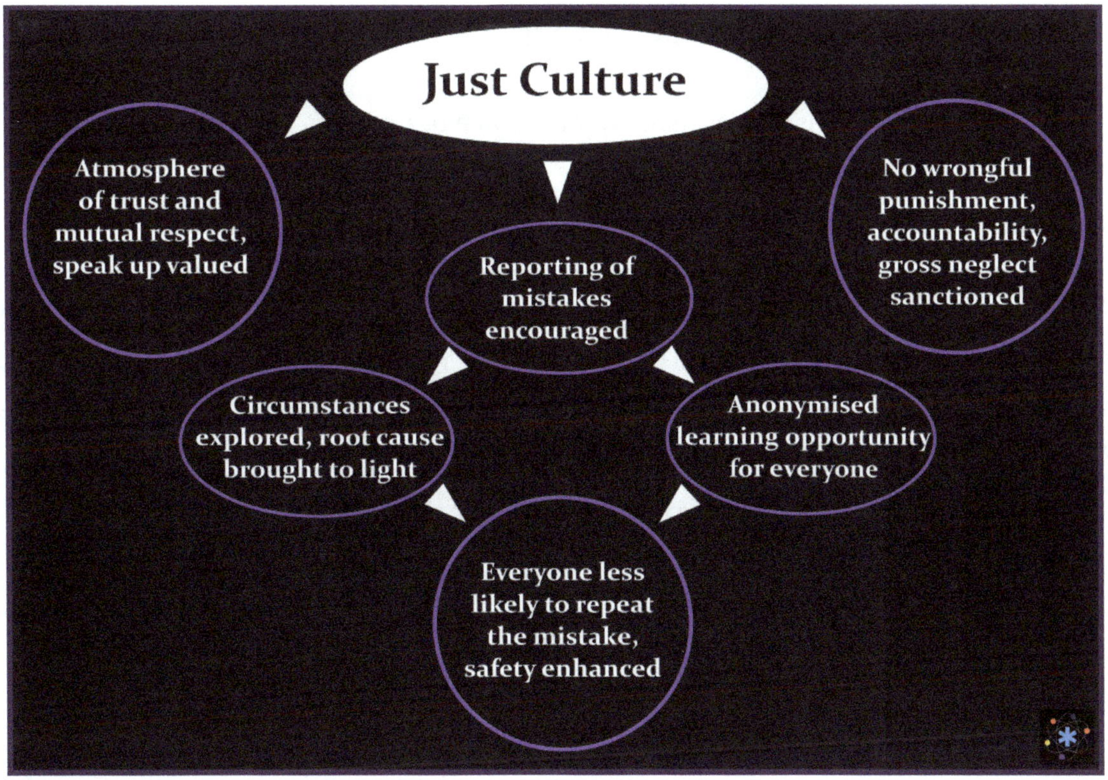

Figure 8: The effects of just culture

10.4. How to Set up a Just Culture

If we want to establish a just culture in our working environment, we benefit from taking the following steps together with our teams:

- we evaluate, what mistakes typically happen
- we continue to look for further errors
- we assess what safety guidelines exist and which ones we want to add
- we establish the boundaries of acceptable behaviour and errors
- we determine, how mistakes are reported and resolved
- we agree on the sanctions that apply to the mistakes according to existing professional frameworks
- we determine, when and how often we will inform everyone about the reported mistakes and the measures we have taken

10.5. How to Make the Success Visible

Success is measurable, which is why we should also make our success using in just culture visible. To achieve this, we need to determine how often we will check the quantity and kinds of the reported mistakes. In addition, we agree on how to assess the success of our measures.

Remember

Our employees have a strong interest in learning about our joint successes. This will keep everyone motivated to continue to contribute to our just culture.

10.6. These Lines of Business Use Just Culture

The following lines of business have adopted just culture from aviation:

The healtcare system uses it in order to avoid mistakes which lead to injuries, illness and death of patients (1). Just culture adds to the enhancement of patient safety.

Maritime shipping applies it to prevent disastrous accidents, in which many people may lose their lives or serious environmental pollution may be caused.

The railroad industry, in which trains with several hundred souls on board are en route on tightly knit networks of tracks on a busy schedule, benefits from just culture as well. Mistakes when working the switches or when signs had been overlooked have had fatal consequences in the past.

10.7. The Comprehensive Summary of Chapter 10

Just culture: no unfounded blame/punishment, accountability in case of guilt, gross negligence is sanctioned as agreed on within the industry/company.

- scapegoating and punishment of all types of errors lead to a cover-up of mistakes
- => important opportunities for learning and enhancing safety through changes are lost
- a non-punitive culture even resulted in repeated risky behaviour and inferior outcomes

- just culture was established as the right balance to deal with errors and negligence
- main features: clearly defined tasks and responsibilities, anyone can make mistakes, speak up valued, honest reporting of mistakes, circumstances and causes are explored => improvement
- if guilty, people are held accountable, gross negligence may lead to the loss of the professional licence
- the whole team should be involved in a just culture, goals, standards, error reporting system, sanctions according to the industry's framework, measurement of progress needed
- praise your team and celebrate successes together

10.8. Where to Place Just Culture

Just culture is part ot safety culture, with which we will occupy ourselves in the following chapter.

10.9. References

1) GAIN Working Group E (2004) A Roadmap to a Just Culture: Enhancing the Safety Environment. https://flightsafety.org/files/just_culture.pdf, most recently accessed: July 31st, 2023

2) Boysen BG (2013) Just Culture: A Foundation for Balanced Accountability and Patient Safety. The Ochsner Journal 13: 400-406 https://www.ncbi.nlm.nih.gov/pmc/articles/PMC3776518/pdf/i1524-5012-13-3-400.pdf, most recently accessed: July 31st, 2023

11

11. Safety Culture

These Contents Are Waiting for You in the Eleventh Chapter

How do we define safety margins and why do we tend to push them? Why do we need a safety culture and what does it entail? In this chapter, we will reveal why we use the term "culture" and who is part of it. Furthermore, we will look at the five elements which, according to James Reason, constitute our safety culture. Finally, we will explore how much a safety culture, as illustrated here, is appreciated around the world in correlation with the prevailing type of hierarchy.

11.1. Mistakes and Safety Margins

11.1.1. Human Factors Constantly Threaten Our Work

The human factors inevitably influence all of our work, no matter how hard we try to avoid them (1, 2). We all know what a lack of time and resources feels like. There might also be a lack of appropriate equipment, or training. Showing assertiveness and speaking up is not always easy, either. Consequently, we all make mistakes, mostly involuntarily, regardless of our rank in the company. We have already examined how to deal with them using threat and error management (TEM) (chapter 7). In addition, we have taken a look at just culture in order to learn how to create a culture in which we can report errors and risks without fear of unfair punishment (chapter 10).

11.1.2. What Happens if Safety Margins Are Being Pushed?

What Are Safety Margins?

We establish safety margins by employing crew resource management principles wisely. For example, we use checklists, we crosscheck with colleagues, and we use certain communication techniques to enhance the safety of our work.

Remember

The purpose of safety margins is to create a possibility to detect and correct errors, before they cause any harm.

Why Are Safety Margins Likely to Be Pushed?

We all know that there are time pressure and the need to work cost-effectively at almost any workplace. Thus, cutting corners might be all too tempting, even in high-risk work environments, such as aviation or healthcare.

How Are Safety Margins Being Pushed?

Pitfall

An Example From Aviation: Leaving out Important Steps During Maintenance

During the maintenance work on the aircraft N233YV, a Raytheon (Beechcraft) 1900D, which was used on Air Midwest Flight 5481 from Charlotte-Douglas International Airport, North Carolina, to Greenville-Spartanburg International Airport, Greer, South Carolina, USA, on 8 January 2003, several crucial steps had been left out (3).

Following that, the elevator (used to lift or lower the nose of the plane) could not be operated at its full range of movement, which contributed to the crash that happened on that flight.

Pitfall

An Example From the Emergency Medical Service: Equipment Not Properly Checked

Imagine an ambulance crew which starts a night shift and does not check all the equipment according to the standard operating procedures and checklists. During a call, a patient needs to be intubated, and the light of the laryngoscope, an instrument which is needed to look at the vocal chords and to insert the tube into the trachea, is weak and suddenly goes out.

Now, hectic searching for spare equipment ensues, putting the patient at a serious risk as the procedure of securing his or her airway is delayed.

Possible Consequences of the Pitfalls

Leaving out steps in the maintenance of an airliner, or not checking ambulance equipment properly before a shift are only two examples of pushing the boundaries and, therefore, reducing the safety margins. This might work a few times, encouraging some professionals to push the boundaries even further over time. However, in the end, a potentially fatal disaster is likely to happen.

Remember

The mistakes, which we all make from time to time and the habit of not respecting safety margins both illustrate the need to establish a healthy safety culture.

Like an umbrella, this spans all our efforts to minimise the risk of mistakes and to enhance the safety of our work.

11.2. Safety Culture Is Superordinated to All Efforts to Enhance Safety

11.2.1. Definition

The term "culture" expresses that this is no single concept which is learned during a short term training course. Rather, safety culture consists of beliefs, behaviours, and attitudes towards safety. In addition, the willingness to report and learn from mistakes, as well as flexibility play a role, as we will discover below. Of course, the values and customs of the respective nation and the standards in the line of business influence the safety culture we create or maintain at our respective workplaces.

11.2.2. Who Is Part of Our Safety Culture?

The CEO of any company or business should act as a good example and is responsible for the implementation and maintenance of a healthy safety culture across the entire company or business. All senior managers play a decisive role in supervising, teaching and informing all employees. Last but not least, all employees, who carry out work which involves any risk should be encouraged, to develop and maintain a safety culture awareness. This means that they should actively report mistakes and safety risks, amongst others.

11.2.3. Safety Culture Cannot Be Replaced

Superordinating our safety culture means that it cannot be replaced by existing human factor training, CRM principles and their use, or maintenance resource management (MRM). It is the umbrella under which we carry out anything with respect to enhancing the safety of our business.

A safety management system (SMS) which encompasses all necessary procedures, organisational structures and responsibilities, as well as a reporting system, should be in place (4).

11.3. The Components of a Safety Culture

Several different components make up the safety culture of an organisation. First, we will elucidate which ones James Reason considered crucial. Then, we will examine the influence which, for example, responsibility, leadership, and attitude have.

11.3.1. The Postulate of James Reason

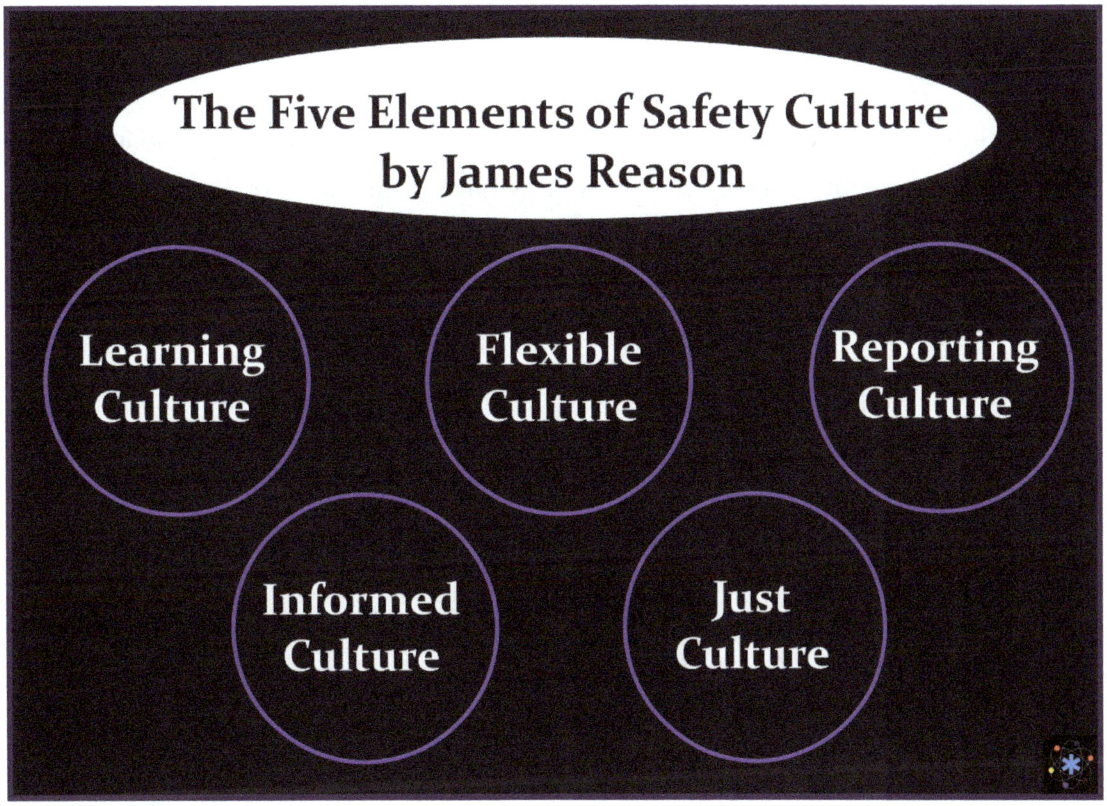

Figure 9: Safety culture

As we can see in the illustration above, James Reason has denominated five elements, which together create a safety culture. Let's take a closer look at how they are defined.

Learning Culture

A company or organisation must be willing to learn from the errors it detects using its reporting system and make the necessary changes. Moreover, each employee needs to understand the safety management system, its processes and continuous improvement.

Informed Culture

Everyone involved in implementing and maintaining a safety culture and acting according to it, knows the principles, attitudes, expected behaviours, and procedures. Data about safety is continuously gathered and assessed, any information about safety is distributed to everyone concerned in a timely manner.

Flexible Culture

The workforce within a company or an organisation is capable of adapting to changing demands or reacting to threats. Sometimes, in this process hierarchies are flattened.

Just Culture

The entire workforce reports mistakes and is not punished wrongfully. Those who are to blame for a mistake, are held accountable after the circumstances have been clarified. If there was gross neglect involved, sanctions, on which the organisation or company has agreed, will be applied, including the loss of a professional licence in accordance with existing guidelines.

Reporting Culture

Employees are encouraged to report mistakes or any safety concerns. The team, or whoever is in charge, then explores the root cause of the mistakes or hazards to safety and works out how to prevent future errors, or how to mitigate the hazards.

11.3.2. The Following Add to the Five Elements

Leadership

Every superior needs to exert leadership and be a good example of how to behave with a true safety culture awareness. This means not pushing safety margins, admitting and correcting own errors, as well as not letting the mistakes of others, a lack of safety culture awareness, or risks go unnoticed. True leaders show the courage to address these errors and risks and hearten their employees to make amendments.

Responsibility

Leaders, but also all employees, are responsible to personally understand the safety management system and the reporting system the company has established.

Attitude and Commitment

Everyone in a company or an organisation who carries out tasks which entail risks, needs to understand what professional attitude is required. Furthermore, the more these employees commit themselves to actively contribute to the safety culture, the better this culture can be, ensuring safe operations.

Communication and Trust

Every company has its own procedures to communicate errors and risks. There should be an atmosphere in which employees can trust their employers that no unjust punishment awaits them if they have made an unintentional error and report it. Communication and trust pertain especially to just culture and reporting culture.

Training

Continuous training courses are provided by many organisations in healthcare, and all companies and organisations involved in aviation. These regular courses deal with human factors, crew resource management, or maintenance resource management. Moreover, at least new employees need to learn about the safety management system, the overall safety culture of a company and how to report errors and risks.

11.4. The Recognition of Safety Culture Is Not the Same Around the World

Hierarchy and the safety culture described in this chapter are interrelated. In countries with a strict hierarchy, for instance, Taiwan, Japan, and Russia, ideas such as the speak up are less common. Thus, certain components of a modern safety culture may not be appreciated as much as they are in a country with a flat hierarchy, such as the USA, Scandinavia, or Ireland.

What shall we do if safety culture is not valued and someone, who is reporting a mistake, is simply dismissed due to "gross neglect" even if the mistake was made unintentionally? Unfortunately, this still happens around the world.

Pause and Think

What steps do you suggest to mend the situation?

What could you do at your own workplace in case you notice room for improvement there?

Concerning the latter, how would you assess your prospects of change?

11.5. The Comprehensive Summary of Chapter 11

Due to inevitable errors and our tendency to push the safety margins, we need a safety culture.

- safety margins help us to detect and correct errors before they cause any harm
- the mentioned pitfalls as examples of how safety margins are being pushed show us what behaviours to avoid in order to prevent a potentially fatal outcome
- safety culture is the umbrella which spans all of our efforts to enhance safety
- J. Reason described five elements: flexible culture, informed culture, just culture, reporting culture, learning culture, also emphasising the term "culture"
- in addition to the five elements we need: leadership, responsibility, attitude, commitment, communication, trust, training
- safety culture is especially appreciated in countries which also have flat hierarchies, such as the USA, the Scandinavian countries, and Ireland
- we still have a long way ahead of us if we want to implement a safety culture or improve an existing one, including an accepted safety management system, and measuring the results of our efforts
- once more, we should praise our teams for great achievements and celebrate our successes

11.6. Read the Next Chapter Whenever It Suits You

In Advent, it is time to create some delicious baked goods. No matter, whether you will be working in the kitchen together with your family, close friends, or within a charity organisation, you will be surprised, how much about crew resource management you have already learned.

11.7. References

1) https://skybrary.aero/articles/human-factors-dirty-dozen, most recently accessed: July 31st, 2023

2) Mellema, GM, Cuevas, HM, Esser, DA, Conway, B, Frisinger, SL (2021) Application of Dupont's Dirty Dozen Framework to Commercial Aviation Maintenance Incidents. International Journal of Aviation Research 13(1): 43-62

3) National Transportation Safety Board, NTSB (2004) Aircraft Accident Report, Loss of Pitch Control During Takeoff, Air Midwest Flight 5481, Raytheon (Beechcraft) 1900D, N233YV, Charlotte, North Carolina, January 8, 2003, https://reports.aviation-safety.net/2003/20030108-0_B190_N233YV.pdf, most recently accessed: July 27th, 2023

4) Stroeve S, Smeltink J, Kirwan B (2022) Assessing and Advancing Safety Management in Aviation. Safety 8: 20. https://doi.org/10.3390/safety8020020 , most recently accessed: August 4th, 2023

12

12. CRM Principles in Your pre-Christmas Kitchen

These Contents Are Waiting for You in the Twelfth Chapter

From the planning stage to superb results, we will look at all the steps it takes to successfully produce delicious baked goods in Advent. As we go along, we will discover where we can use CRM principles to our advantage. Please enjoy the read.

12.1. How to Apply CRM Principles During Your First Preparations

12.1.1. Your Project and First Decisions

The pre-Christmas period demands that you take care of various preparations for Christmas on top of your everyday work. In addition, delicious baked goods are sought after. Now, your presence in the kitchen is required, no matter whether you get down to business there together with your family, your friends, or within a charity organisation.

Already your first considerations demand that you **make decisions**. With whom will you work together? What type of Christmas biscuits or other baked goods are you planning to make? What do you need to shop where, and how will you schedule your work?

12.1.2. Your Team and Further Resources

As you already know, you have got your **team** and further **resources** at your disposal. In your case, these are the possibilities to procure the ingredients, the ingredients themselves, and your fully equipped kitchen.

Skilfully, you use your team during the first preparations and discuss how to **manage the first part of the workload**. Who will buy what? Will you be needing additional equipment, you do not possess in your kitchen? Who could bring it?

12.1.3. Automatically, You Apply CRM Principles in Your Preliminary Discussion

You decide jointly, what kinds of biscuits or fruit loaf you want to bake. Using **closed communication loops**, you repeat once more, what you have decided in order to make sure that you have understood correctly, and everyone means the same.

12.1.4. Shopping Lists and Recipes Resemble Further CRM Principles

With so many ingredients, which you have to purchase in certain quantities, it is, naturally, difficult for you to remember everything by heart. Hence, you write shopping lists, which you have at hand much like **checklists** when you do the shopping. You can look items up at any time and make sure that you don't forget anything.

As you produce your collection of recipes, you are proud, and rightly so. Some recipes have been a success for generations. Other ones you have written down and refined yourself. Your recipes are not mere lists. Rather, they contain additional work instructions. They are your s**tandard operating procedures (SOPs)** so to speak, which help you to carry out all steps according to the guidance in the right order.

Remember

Even before you took your first step into the kitchen, you made decisions, and put together your team, took care of resources, and managed the workload, communicated, used checklists, and arranged your SOPs.

12.2. In medias res, CRM Principles in Your Kitchen

12.2.1. The Kick-Off

In the case we will look at here, there are now you yourself, a close friend of yours and several children gathered in the kitchen. With military precision, **you organise the space first** and make sure that everyone **knows the work environment**. You arrange the ingredients and your equipment. Then, you discuss how to use which of the work tops, and where to put the baking trays, as well as the biscuit tins for your elaborate pieces.

12.2.2. Getting Started With a Well-Managed Workload

As you are going to make several types of biscuits, you discuss with your friend as **team leaders**, who is going to make which. The children as your **team members** will assist you actively and **take on all tasks**, they are already able to perform. Whoever has a question, will ask those at any time, since you are a well-rehearsed and strong team.

12.2.3. How to Carry out Your Teamwork Safely

A long, but cosy afternoon within a familiar group in the kitchen is a safe thing, isn't it? However, aren't there the hot oven and baking trays? The pot with boiling water to peel the almonds? The food processor with perfectly sharpened blades to chop the nuts?

Together you agree on your **safety standards**. These include, for instance, that you not only switch off the food processor, but also disconnect it before anyone is allowed to reach into it.

12.2.4. Your Situational Awareness as an Important CRM Principle Is Required

As you are now baking several kinds of biscuits simultaneously as a **team**, your continuous **situational awareness** is required. **Spatially**, you have to keep an overview of what is being processed, or put where. As **team leaders** you monitor, what steps your **team members** are carrying out at the moment. **Considering time**, superb coordination is necessary.

You keep an eye on your **resources**, i.e. ingredients, recipes, as well as your equipment and apply all of those wisely. Last but not least, the children should not eat too much of the raw dough. To nibble on some of it is allowed, but no one should feel seriously sick.

12.3. Should We Really Add so Much Salt?

12.3.1. The CRM Principle of a Speak up Is Always Important

In the middle of the preparation of a dough, your friend stops herself and utters: "Here it says: 'Two tablespoons of sugar comma salt'". Do the two tablespoons really pertain to the salt as well?" After this **speak up** you stop working immediately.

12.3.2. As a Team You Solve the Problem

As a **team**, you ponder how plausible two tablespoons of salt in a recipe would be. In your opinion, the possibility that this may lead to a good result is limited. Therefore, you **decide** to add a pinch of salt first and then to taste the dough. You could still add more salt later if necessary. The tasting reveals that you have solved the problem well having **discussed it as a team**. The result is perfect.

The original version of this episode had turned out less advantageously. When two students upon the instruction "two tablespoons of sugar, salt" in a recipe for a kaiserschmarrn (a sweet pancake dish) decided to use this quantity on both ingredients, their freshly baked, fluffy kaiserschmarrn was, unfortunately, inedible.

12.4. Flops, Failures, and Fumbles - How to Use CRM Principles Now

As your little daughter separates the eggs, one egg yolk falls into the egg white. Immediately, she visibly saddened **reports** her **mishap** and affirms that she did not do it on purpose. You calm your young assistant and tell her that it was right to **inform you about it** so quickly. Moreover, you tell her **that you are not angry with her** in perfect accordance with just culture (chapter 10).

After you managed to recover the egg yolk with a large tablespoon, **you bring the cause of the mistake to light**. Your daughter is not trained well enough yet to separate the eggs safely under the time pressure she just felt. You promise her to practise together with her the next time you bake a cake. For now, **you assign an easier task to her**, which is just as important, namely, to cut out the shapes of the mini gingerbread men.

12.5. Highly Concentrated at Work

12.5.1. A Sterile Kitchen?

You are in the middle of your project. On a tight schedule, you put new baking trays into your oven. After only ten minutes, other ones have to be removed from the oven, stored and then processed further. Still, you as a team work on different kinds of Christmas biscuits simultaneously.

Maximum concentration is the order of the day. Thus, **you direct** the **communication** within your team entirely to your **work.** Right now, you have no time for remarks like "Have you seen the four metre tall Christmas tree, the Joneses have bought?"

You have almost established a "sterile kitchen rule" in analogy to the sterile cockpit rule (during times of highly concentrated work, only issue-related items are discussed and executed) (1, 2). Automatically, you refrain from other actions, which have nothing to do with the actual baking process, such as eating or talking on the phone.

12.5.2. Praise Does Not Belong to the CRM Principles (Yet)

In spite of your concentrated work, you do not forget to **praise your team members**, whenever they have executed a task well: "You have cut out the shapes of the mini gingerbread men beautifully. I am proud of you." You instinctively feel how important this recognition is for everyone in the **team** (chapter 1). All members lean in even more.

12.6. You Are Enjoying Your Success - in the Truest Sense of the Word

Many working hours lie behind **you and your team**. Exhausted, but happy you are sitting around the dinner table. For dessert, a small plate of the freshly baked biscuits is served.

Almost automatically, a conversation about the afternoon starts, which nearly resembles a **debriefing** of your jointly executed work. You remember, for example, the two tablespoons of salt with amusement and decide to explore such **uncertainties** always **as a team** in the future.

Top Tip

Once again, you praise your industrious companions, and rightly so, because you have every reason to be proud of your work!

12.7. The Concise Explanation of the CRM Terms Used in This Chapter

In Table 2 below, you will find all the CRM terms used above (printed in bold type) along with a brief explanation. Amongst them, and, of course, explained in the table, is the first of the 15 CRM Key Points, which we will examine in-depth in volume 2 of this Special CRM Collection:

The 15 CRM Key Points

1. Know the environment.

Table 2 The CRM Terms Used in Chapter 12 at a Glance

CRM Term	Explanation
team	team leader, team members, their combined knowledge, skills, and attitude all members are also resources
team leader	overview over all tasks, and pieces of information, decisions, and results distributes the tasks, oversees the execution and completion of all tasks guides and supports team members, encourages speak ups and constructive suggestions
team members	take on all tasks they are capable of, report the completion of tasks to the team leader they ask their questions and possess the assertiveness to speak up or make suggestions
resources	all team members and their abilities, all pieces of information, equipment, help from other teams
checklists	contain all items which may not be left out during a certain procedure
SOPs	comprise all necessary steps to execute a task, SOPs often include in what case the respective task needs to be performed, who should do what, and, sometimes, in what dedicated area or room the action should take place (e.g., emergency room)
communication	our communication should always be clear, concise, and calm communication techniques encompass: standardised phraseology, closed communication loops, and the sterile cockpit rule, see below
closed communication loops	the receiver of a message repeats what the sender said => it is clarified whether everything is understood correctly, the sender listens carefully and corrects as necessary
sterile cockpit rule	during certain phases of the flight, only communication pertaining to the tasks at hand is permitted, no private or other topics may be discussed
knowing the work environment	this first of the 15 CRM Key Principles by Rall and Gaba emphasises how important it is to know how the workplace is organised and where all the resources are
organising the workspace	a clear layout helps in stressful situations, see also "know the work environment" an organised workspace helps to prevent unnecessary mistakes and delays, which, in turn, could cause stress and trigger (further) errors
safety standards	part of the safety management system, measures and procedures enhancing work safety
workload management	the workload should be distributed appropriately amongst the team members, also taking their current state of abilities into account phases with a low workload should be used to prepare for those with a tight schedule preparations even allow for extra time to deal with unexpected occurrences

Table 2 continues on the next page.

CRM Terms	Explanation
decision-making	teams must make sound decisions, also when stressed, taking all the facts and possible outcomes, as well as their resources, into account it helps to use standardised decision-making models, such as FORDEC and TDODAR
situational awareness, five levels	there are five levels of situational awareness, from "tuned out" (e.g. lying on the beach) over "relaxed" (driving in light traffic), "focused" (driving on an icy road), "high alert" (downhill racing) to "comatose" (not able to react appropriately any more due to a startling event) switching between levels 2 and 3 is suitable for many tasks and can be maintained for the longest time span by comparison
situational awareness, various areas	spatially, one needs to be aware where one is (e.g. when flying at night without any visible references), and where the resources are (e.g. in the emergency medical service: where the nearest suitable hospital is) concerning time: how much is left for a task, are we on schedule resources: what resources have we got, where are they, how can we obtain them there is also technical situational awareness, and regarding information taken together, it is the awareness of the situation as a whole, which we need to consider when, for instance, making decisions, or reflecting on a desired outcome
speak up	any team member may speak up if he or she has noticed a threat or a mistake, or has a concern the speak up should always be explored by the team
report a mishap and adequate reaction	the atmosphere within a team should encourage everyone to report a mishap the reaction should be adequate, just culture should be applied, see below
bringing the cause of an error to light	we see an error at the surface, but we need to find its root cause in order to prevent it in the future
just culture	no wrongful punishment, causes of errors and all circumstances need to be explored in case of guilt, one is held accountable for the mistake made in case of gross negligence, one is sanctioned according to the standards of the industry
debriefing	after an action, the entire team discusses what went well and what needs improvement the newest team members should speak first, so the experienced hear their real views the root causes of potentially made errors should be explored constructively
praise for a process, or a well-executed task	praise for a process helps us to understand why we achieved something and to repeat or even build on our successes

12.8. The Comprehensive Summary of Chapter 12

Pause and Think Before You Read the Summary

Where will you apply what you have read in this chapter?

No matter where we work as a team, we will always profit from using CRM principles.

- the teamwork starts with the preparations, as does the use of CRM
- already during planning, we need resources, communicate with our team members, and apply checklists and SOPs
- we need to know the environment, organise the workspace, and establish safety measures
- we act as team leaders and team members, we distribute the workload and speak up
- when something goes wrong, we use CRM and just culture to explore the root causes of the error and deal with it according to the agreed standards
- when the workload is high, we concentrate on our tasks and refrain from speaking of other topics or addressing matters which are not related to our work
- praise for a process or a well-executed task is always important and motivates us to lean in
- as a team, we should hold a constructive debriefing session when we are finished

12.9. If You Would Like to Follow Me...

... to the preview of Volume 2 on page 137. There, you will find the scope of the important, but also compelling topics we will explore next in this Special CRM Collection. I hope to welcome you back to another illuminating read.

12.10. References

1) Code of Federal Regulations, § 121.542. Flight crewmembers duties (last amended 2/08/2023) https://www.ecfr.gov/current/title-14/chapter-I/subchapter-G/part-121/subpart-T/section-121.542, most recently accessed: August 7th, 2023

2) Landsberg B. (2000) The Sterile Cockpit. https://www.aopa.org/news-and-media/all-news/2000/june /pilot/the-sterile-cockpit, most recently accessed: August 7th, 2023

Preview of the Next Volume

In the second volume of the Special CRM Series, we will start with the human factors as summarised in the so-called "Dirty Dozen". We will look at them one by one to become aware of them first, before we discover what CRM principles help us to minimise their impact on our work.

At crash sites and dangerous workplaces it is crucial to maximise scene safety. We will discuss the techniques that help us to work as safely as possible even if we encounter violence at a scene. Knife attacks in public are a particularly atrocious form of violence at the scene. Unfortunately, they happen more and more often, at least in Germany. Hence, we will elucidate how professionals and lay persons can prepare for such an event and how they can act in the best possible manner.

How do we conduct structured debriefing sessions constructively after one of our emergency calls? How does such a debriefing differ from the one we hold after completing a scenario during simulation training? Using examples from the emergency medical service, we will answer these questions. In addition, we will reveal how we overcome obstacles to debriefing sessions in our daily routine. Last but not least, we will highlight, how we transfer our learning points into our work and how to offer them to our colleagues.

What are the main characteristics of post-traumatic stress (PTS) and a post-traumatic stress disorder (PTSD)? How do we distinguish them and which of those needs treatment? Why is it so important to be honest about these conditions? We will shed light on this vital theme and also explore an extraordinary example of courage and openness.

The 15 CRM Key Points by Rall and Gaba transfer many a crucial aspect of CRM into medical teamwork. These 15 concise points are as easily comprehensible as they are beneficial. We will examine them one at a time, before we playfully highlight their use.

Appendix 1: Two Unique Cheat Sheets

How to Apply New CRM or Any Knowledge in Practice

The transfer of new knowledge starts at the very beginning of planned educational activities.

Whenever you buy CRM learning material or enrol in a training course: What is your aim?

- What is the status quo in your team and what would you like to learn?
- Who could support you? If you attend as a team: What do you want to achieve together?
- During reading/training: Where in your work can you use what you have just learned?

It is all about your will to change something. It is your responsibility, but also a great opportunity for you, to apply your new knowledge actively to achieve the envisioned change.

Depending on your role in the team, the following might help to make the desired changes:

- As a team leader: Involve your team. Ask open questions about their suggestions (open questions start with "what", "why", or "how" in order not to restrict the answer right from the start).
- As a team member: Talk to your colleagues and your team leader (if applicable) about why you want to learn more about CRM, what the contents will be, and the benefits you expect for the entire team and — last but not least — for your patients, customers, or particular outcomes.
- Everyone when discussing within the team: Support your suggestions with examples from your experience, as well as references. Ask others to share their ideas, but also their concerns. Respond with open questions to ideas and concerns to further explore them.
- Everyone: Help to create an atmosphere of learning and mutual constructive support.

A Secret From CRM Training

Use the power of silence after a question. Let the other person take time to think before answering.

Whenever you use new knowledge to make changes, either alone or with your team, use this cycle:

- define your goals, make sure that they are achievable, include how to measure your success
- plan the necessary steps and a timeline, consider all your resources
- carry out your plan, observe the effects of your efforts as you proceed
- evaluate your achievements, assess successes and necessary improvements
- restart the cycle

Gaining the Confidence to Speak up

There are still major issues we need to address when talking about the speak up:

At some workplaces, and by some of our colleagues, speak ups are not valued yet. Time and again, professionals do not dare to speak up due to fear of punishment, or damage to their career prospects, or to a relationship. Moreover, they might not want to hurt anyone's feelings, or to be "alone on one side" whilst all others in the team either remain silent, or do not see the threat or error.

It is important to break the silence of bystanders caused by group dynamics: If in a group, people tend to wait and see what others will do. If the others do not speak up, those in the group who hesitate, become also more likely to refrain from it.

If we have spoken up, but the other person does not consider our point, we must respect his or her will if only this person is concerned. If others are in danger, we should dare to insist.

The following might help, depending on how urgent the situation is:

- the accident in Tenerife and its effects on CRM training should clearly illustrate the value of a speak up
- we should state precisely why we are concerned about the patient's safety/the flight/the result and that our speak up is not about ourselves, let alone about criticism
- if time permits and if applicable, we should introduce ourselves and mention our role
- we should work out a structure for our speak ups: what threat or error we have noticed, what consequences we expect, what our suggestion is, and, lastly, we ask what others think
- we should also speak up when someone is pushing the safety margins, as this may lead to an unfavourable outcome, meaning that careless behaviour and subsequent errors reach the patient, the safety of a flight, or the famous bottom line
- if in acute danger, there might only be time for a quick "stop", "watch out", etc.

Remember

Taken together, we can only continue our work on our own speak ups (confidence and technique), and on convincing the ones around us of the necessity and the value of speak ups. Of course, we should praise those with whom we have established speak ups successfully.

Appendix 2: Sources of Further Information

Depending on your line of business, your personal interests, and the way in which you use CRM in your professional life, you might find the following resources helpful. Of course, this is a selection, you might as well know other valuable publications and websites.

1. CRM and Safety in Aviation, General Information on Aviation

Books

Kanki BG, Anca J, Chidester TR, Editors (2019) Crew Resource Management (3rd edition). Academic Press, an Imprint of Elsevier, London, Oxford, Cambridge, San Diego

US Department of Transportation, Federal Aviation Administration (2016) Pilots′ Handbook of Aeronautical Knowledge. Aviation Supplies & Academics, Inc., Newcastle, Washington

Resources Online

The Skybrary has information on almost any aeronautical topic: https://skybrary.aero/

Dailymotion.com offers a myriad of quality air crash investigation documentaries:

https://www.dailymotion.com/

National and International Aviation and Safety Authorities (Selection)

Australian Transportation Safety Bureau (ATSB): https://www.atsb.gov.au/

Civil Aviation Authority (CAA), UK: https://www.caa.co.uk/

European Union Aviation Safety Agency (EASA) EASA Pro: https://www.easa.europa.eu/en/home

Federal Aviation Administration (FAA): https://www.faa.gov/

International Civil Aviation Organization (ICAO): https://www.icao.int/Pages/default.aspx

International Air Transport Association (IATA): https://www.iata.org

National Transportation Safety Board (NTSB) USA: https://www.ntsb.gov/Pages/home.aspx

2. CRM and Safety in Medicine

A Recommended Book About Simulation Debriefing

Oriont D, Guillaume A, (2018) Pocket Book for Simulation Debriefing in Healthcare. Springer International Publishing AG, Cham, Switzerland

Patient Safety and Reporting of Critical Incidences in Medicine

Using the following link of the National Health Service (NHS), UK, many themes concerning patient safety and safety culture are accessible: https://www.england.nhs.uk/patient-safety/report-patient-safety-incident/

Simulation in Medicine

Society for Simulation in Europe (SESAM): https://www.sesam-web.org/

Society for Simulation in Healthcare (SSH): https://www.ssih.org/

Dear Readers

Congratulations!

First of all, huge praise to all of you who have worked your way through this book so diligently to explore ideas and acquire new knowledge.

Keep Going!

When you use CRM as you carry out your routine work, what changes do you notice? How can you use your observations to enhance your and your team's success?

Your Comments and Reviews Are Highly Appreciated

Just as important as your using CRM actively are your thoughts on this book. What did you like? What are your suggestions? Of course, you can also ask your questions. I would truly appreciate your comments. If you like to provide a review of this book, I would be delighted. You will find all the necessary information at:

https://www.communicatio-optima.com/celebration-rewards-comments-and-reviews

You can also use the form on my homepage, subchapter 7:

https://www.communicatio-optima.com/en

A Reward for Your Hard Work

As you have studied so hard using this book, there is a reward waiting for you. You can claim it on the page mentioned above. There, you will find a description of all the items you can choose from. These include informative CRM articles, as well as articles on writing and self-publishing. You do not have to leave a comment or provide a review in order to collect your reward.

For now, I wish you every success with your teamwork!

Yours sincerely,

Eva-Maria Schottdorf

About the Author

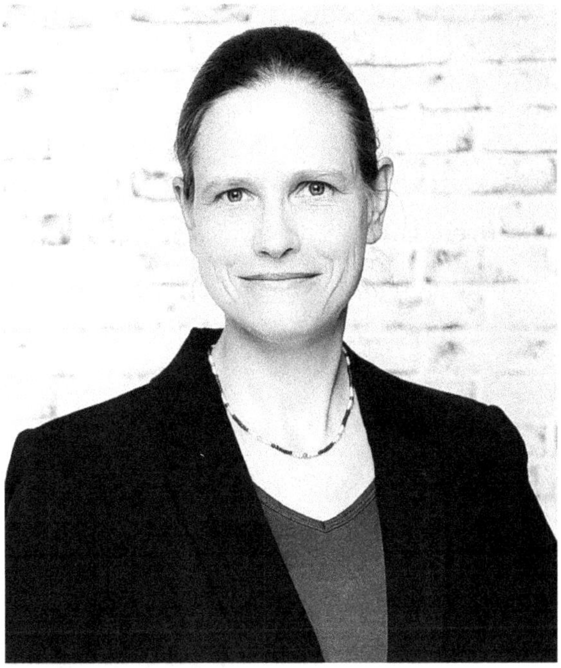

Eva-Maria Schottdorf, Author-Publisher
Portrait: Studioline, Munich, Germany

Dr. Eva-Maria Schottdorf has worked as a freelance prehospital emergency physician in Germany, Austria, and Switzerland for more than ten years. She is a certified trainer for crew resource management (CRM), which originated in aviation, and uses its concepts during her emergency calls.

As she loves flying, be it to international conferences or to explore new destinations, she has made a point of obtaining a CRM Trainer Certificate which is recognised by the European Union Aviation Safety Agency (EASA). In addition, she has trained as a doc on board in order to help voluntarily in case of an in-flight emergency.

As an author-publisher and seminar trainer, she is passionate about passing on the successful concepts of CRM to committed professionals, not only from high-risk work environments. For more information on the author and her work, please visit her website at:

https://www.communicatio-optima.com

What Is the Work of a Self-Publishing Author Like?

Being a self-publishing author makes it possible to retain all rights to one's book if one uses one's own International Standard Book Numbers (ISBNs). In addition, one takes care of the book from the first draft until its publication. A self-publishing author makes all decisions, ranging from design to sales. The author is never alone, but hires services such as editing and proofreading.

Eva-Maria Schottdorf not only finds it really exciting to pursue such a varied career, but she has also discovered along her way that non-fiction authors need specific knowledge when publishing and marketing their books. As she loves to pass on her skills in order to help others with their projects, she has been offering consulting for non-fiction authors since March 2024. You can read all about it on the following page:

https://www.communicatio-optima.com/en/consulting-for-textbook-authors/

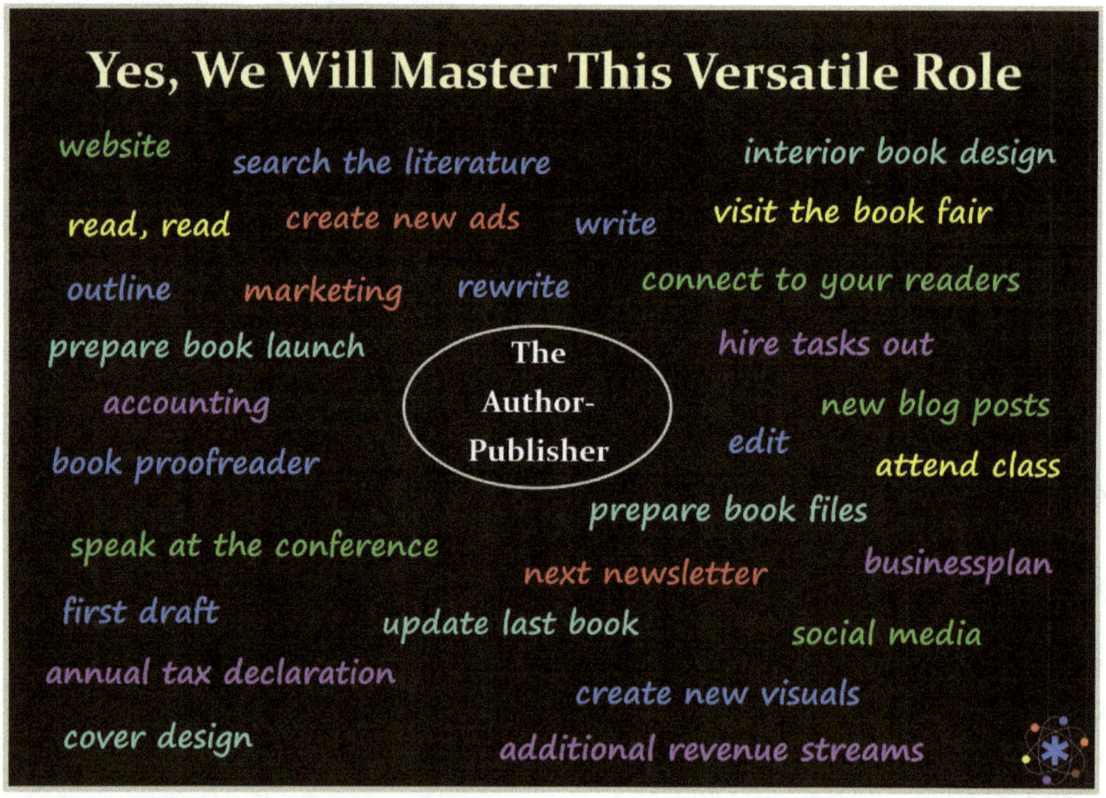

Not only the actual writing belongs to the exciting career of a self-publishing author.

CRM Glossary

Below, you will find all the CRM terms explained, which you encounter in this book. A "=>" before a term in the explanation tells you that this term is also listed in the glossary. Some of them appear in the Medical or the Aeronautical Glossary.

10-for-10 concept: A team performs a team time out, which lasts a few seconds to decide what to do during the next ten minutes, when it has diagnosed a problem. All members interrupt what they are doing, and the team uses a structured approach: Problem? Team? Facts? Plan the steps. Distribute the workload. Questions? When there are no more questions, the team acts as planned.

Chain of events: A chain of events summarises all the events which contributed to an incident or accident. The events can happen one after another or at the same time. They are typically intertwined with each other.

Checklist: A checklist contains all necessary steps of a procedure. If the order in which the steps need to occur is crucial, the checklist is presented in this order. In aviation, there are three types of checklists: 1. **Read and Verify**, usually performed from memory. The actual checklist is only consulted to ensure that no step has been left out. 2. **Challenge and Response**, one team member asks another about a certain item, and the second member responds and states whether the item has been carried out or not, or whether it needs improvement. 3. **Read and Do**, these are for emergencies in aviation.

Crew resource management (CRM): In aviation, the crew (compriising cockpit and cabin crew) manages its => resources in a way that enhances flight safety and prevents mistakes. As not all errors can be avoided due to => the human factors, the team uses several techniques to detect them, before they do any harm. In other lines of business, teams manage their respective resources with the same goals.

CRM development in six generations: Many parties were (and still are) involved in the development of CRM. They include airlines, pilots, investigators, aviation experts, universities, and => civil aviation authorities. The collaboration between them and even between competing airlines, is unique. In the 1970s, the first generation was called cockpit resource management. It was followed by the second generation and now called crew resource management as it now included the cabin crew. The first two generations aimed at error prevention in the first place. The subsequent generations were: 3.: The focus was more on CRM than on error prevention. 4.: Advanced training methods were introduced. 5.: Back to error prevention. 6.: Introduction of => threat and error management (TEM) and => line oriented safety audits (LOSA).

Communication in CRM: The communication at high-risk workplaces needs to be precise and unmistakable. Thus, several communication techniques have been elaborated, such as the => sterile cockpit rule, => closed communication loops, => standardised phraseology, and the => speak up.

Closed communication loops: What a team member has said is repeated by the recipient of a message. This is vital, as the sender of the message can check whether everything is correct. In case of a misunderstanding, a correction is possible.

Debriefing session: A fulfilled task, an incident, or a simulation exercise are followed by such a session during which a team reflects on the actions, the communication, the events, and the outcome in a structured manner. It is important to find the causes behind errors, but also those behind a great success.

Decision-making: A team has to make many decisions, sometimes in at first chaotic circumstances, or in a short time span. Decision-making describes the process from gathering the facts, analysing them, considering the resources, the risks and the potential outcomes, before the actual decision is made. => Decision-making models help a team to structure this process and to remember the important steps.

Decision-making models: These models enhance safety as they help a team, especially in stressful situations, to consider all relevant information when it makes its decision. Common decision-making models are => FORDEC and => TDODAR.

Dirty Dozen: This is a well-known summary of common => human factors and includes: lack of knowledge, lack of teamwork, lack of communication, lack of resources, lack of assertiveness, lack of awareness, pressure, norms, complacency, stress, fatigue, and distraction.

Error: An error occurs when someone has done something wrong, or has miscommunicated. The error results in a deviation from planned actions, interferes with the expectations of the team or organisation, reduces the => safety margin, and can lead to an adverse event. In addition, the error can develop into a => threat. See also => human errors.

Error chain: The error chain with its eleven links is a concept in aviation, which is used to detect the human factors that have contributed to an accident. The links include: no-one flying the aircraft or monitoring the current state of progress, no-one looking out of the window, ambiguity, distraction/preoccupation, confusion, using any undocumented procedure, violating limitations/regulations, unresolved discrepancies,, failure to meet targets, deviation from SOPs, incomplete communication.

FORDEC: a => decision-making model comprising facts, options, risks, decision, execution, check.

Help: a => resource in => CRM, the team has to decide whether it needs hands or brains. It should know where to find help and call for it early.

Human errors: They cause at least 70% of all accidents. We have to be aware of their existence and the fact that they are inevitable. => CRM provides us with measures to deal with them, ideally before they cause any major harm.

Human factors (HF): There are social HF, such as pressure and norms, HF associated with behaviour, such as "lack of assertiveness" and "complacency", but also cognitive ones, such as "lack of knowledge". All of the HF are inherent in human beings and make us prone to => errors. See also => Dirty Dozen.

Instructor, CRM, simulation: CRM or simulation instructors create the training scenarios and conduct simulator training, which is followed by the crucial => debriefing session. It is most important that they rather facilitate the communication than teach and, through this facilitation, help the team members to detect successes and room for improvements themselves.

Just culture: A culture at a workplace in which errors are handled fairly, without unjust punishment. The mistakes are explored, the circumstances, others who were involved, and contributing factors are addressed. The person who made the mistake has to take responsibility and will be sanctioned according to the standards in the industry. In case of gross negligence, he or she may even lose the professional licence. Just culture is part of => safety culture.

Knowledge, skills, and attitude are the three areas of learning. The hardest one to improve is attitude.

Medical training scenario: With the help of real actors and actresses, or a simulator, a team works its way through a realistic medical case and simulates using all necessary medications and equipment. Whilst gross medical errors are addressed during the => debriefing session, the main focus is on => CRM, => teamwork, and => communication.

Non-punitive or non-blaming culture: This is the opposite of the => punitive or blaming culture, which had prevailed first. In non-punitive culture, employees reported mistakes, but expected not to be punished and blamed the organisation for the errors.

Praise: Not a CRM principle yet, but an important part of a constructive atmosphere in which motivation and encouragement prevail. There is praise for a trait and praise for a process. Using the latter helps team members to understand why they were successful and that they should apply their methods to future tasks.

Punitive or blaming culture preceded the => non-punitive culture. Causes of errors, circumstances, or the ones who had also contributed to the error, were of no particular interest. Rather, one person was blamed and sanctioned, no matter how much he or she had really done wrong.

Resources include the team leader and all team members, their knowledge, skills, and attitude, all available equipment, all pieces of information, as well as => help from other teams.

Safety culture: According to James Reason, it consists of five elements: => just culture, learning culture, reporting culture, informed culture, and flexible culture.

Safety management system (SMS): It is a vital part of => safety culture, as it helps to structure safety management. The SMS, according to the ICAO, encompasses organisational structures, accountabilities, procedures and policies. In addition, the courses of action, which are necessary to achieve and maintain at least acceptable safety standards, are documented.

Safety margin: The distance between the point at which we are and carry out a procedure safely and the circle around this point, which marks the line between safe operations and an undesired outcome. The safety margin is reduced by => threats, the => errors we make, an => undesired aircraft state (UAS) and risks.

Simulation: In simulation training, certain courses of action are rehearsed. Whilst no airliner can crash and no patient can be harmed, the team may repeat the tasks until it can perform them safely, even when stressed. The latter can be trained in particular. The actual training is always followed by a => debriefing session.

Simulation training in aviation: Every pilot has to participate in simulator training regularly. The interior of the simulator is built like an original cockpit of a particular aircraft type. There, certain manoeuvres, such as emergency landings, are practised and debriefed.

Simulation training in medicine is introduced in more and more specialist fields, such as anaesthesia and emergency medicine. A team uses a simulator (a mannequin that can show vital signs, change its complexion, and sometimes even speak) as their patient in a dedicated simulator room. As it performs the anamnesis, makes a diagnosis, and starts treatment, the instructors watch from an adjacent room and videotape the scenario. The observations and the video are then used during the => debriefing session.

Situational awareness: Whenever a team carries out a task, it should be aware of all cues from the surroundings and all pieces of information. **Spatial awareness** includes, for instance, altitude and heading in aviation, and the terrain, or building in the emergency medical service (EMS). **Awareness of the time** means knowing how much time has elapsed, how much is still left, and whether the team is on schedule with its tasks. **Technical awareness** means being aware of all pieces of technical information, the currently available equipment, and the values it indicates.

Speak up: Important part of => communication. Whenever a team leader or team member notices an => error or => threat, he or she should alert the team. Ideally, the team performs a team time out to evaluate the concerns and to determine the best course of action.

Standard operating procedure (SOP): An SOP contains more than the necessary steps of a procedure in the right order like a => checklist does. Reading an SOP, you will also learn who will do what and where the action is supposed to take place. The date of the latest revision is mentioned, as is the date on which the next revision is due.

Standard phraseology: In aviation, but also when EMS professionals communicate on the radio, standardised sentences and phrases are used in order to prevent misunderstandings.

Stress is one => human factor of the => Dirty Dozen. There is acute and chronic stress, hyper- and hypostress, eustress and distress.

TDODAR is a => decision-making model which consists of time, diagnosis, options, decide, act/assign, review. The model was developed in aviation and is used by British Airways, for instance.

Team: It always consists of a => team leader and => team members who exhibit assertiveness. All members bring their => knowledge, skills, and attitude as valuable assets to the team. They may, however, also suffer from a personal stressful condition to name one of the => human factors. As dream teams are made and not born, they should attend => team training together and cultivate a constructive atmosphere for their => teamwork.

Team leader: He or she has an overview of all tasks and information, but also of who is doing what and when tasks need to be finished. The team leader distributes the tasks and helps the => team members if they have any questions.

Team members: The team members carry out the tasks, speak up with assertiveness, and call for a team time out if they feel it is necessary. They report to the => team leader when they have finished a task and are ready to take on a new one. They also state it clearly if a task is too difficult for them so that a team leader can assign it to another member. This is important in order to avoid unnecessary stress and mistakes.

Team training: It is crucial to train together who work together in order to facilitate a smooth workflow during => teamwork and to perfect the => communication and => workload management.

Teamwork: All team members and their leader should understand that the => knowledge, skills, and attitude of everyone counts, whilst they should fit into the team and act in their respective roles at the same time. This ensures that the team works in synergy to achieve great results, even when handling complex tasks.

Threat and error management (TEM): Introduced with the sixth generation of => CRM development, TEM teaches us how to deal with => threats, which come from the outside, and => errors, which a team may make or actually has made.

TEM philosphy: We **anticipate** that errors and threats will inevitably occur and stay vigilant in order to **recognise** them early, which results in **recovery**, i. e. re-establishment of the => safety margins using the appropriate countermeasures.

Threats: Like => errors, threats are inevitable. They come from the outside, the team itself has not made an error. Threats can, however, be the result of an error that another team has made, for instance, in aircraft maintenance before the respective aeroplane is used on a flight. Other threats include factors which we cannot influence, such as weather conditions, or a pitch-dark night.

Workload management: A => team distributes the workload in a way that no-one has too much, too little, or too difficult a task to do. Every => team member reports to the => team leader when a task is finished and he or she is ready to take on a new one.

Medical Glossary

Below, you will find short explanations to all medical terms used in this book. A "=>" before a term within an explanation indicates that it is listed in the glossaries as well.

Adrenaline: A hormone which prepares the body for the => fight or flight response. Amongst other reactions to this hormone, the heart rate is increased, breathing is deeper and faster, the pupils are dilated, the blood glucose level is increased, and blood flows to the muscles rather than to the intestines.

Cortisol: A hormone which is produced by the adrenal glands and usually kept in a fine balance. It regulates the reaction to stress, the glucose metabolism and the blood pressure, and it also reduces inflammation. The cortisol levels are elevated in stressful situations. Whilst this is natural and of no concern in acute stress, which triggers the => fight or flight response, a continuously elevated cortisol level in chronically stressed people harms the body. Symptoms then include weight gain due to a chronically elevated blood sugar level, fragile skin, and acne.

Emergency medical service (EMS): In many countries, acute medical care is provided by ambulance crews, whereas EMS in other countries, for instance, in Germany and Austria, includes prehospital emergency physicians who also travel directly to the scene. Furthermore, helicopter crews, consisting of a pilot, a paramedic, and a doctor, assist, for instance, in the event of a major accident, or when a patient needs to be transported to a specialised hospital further away.

Endorphins are hormones produced by the pituitary gland and the hypothalamus, both areas of the brain, when in stress or pain, but also during, for example, exercise. They reduce pain and enhance the sense of well-being.

FAST: This acronym stands for face (Is the facial expression symmetrical?), arms (Can the patient hold them up?), speech (Does the patient speak clearly and understand what is being said?), and time (When did the symptoms start?). FAST is used to recognise the most common symptoms of a => stroke rapidly.

Fight-or-flight response: The body's response to a startle. We first freeze before we start to fight or flee quickly. => Adrenaline prepares the body for these actions.

Intubation: After general anaesthesia is induced (not necessary during resuscitation), a tube is inserted into the patient's airway to secure it and to ventilate him or her.

Micronutrients: Substances which the body essentially needs in small quantities. They comprise the vitamins A, B, C, D (the skin produces it when exposed to sunlight, but not enough during the winter months), E, and K, as well as minerals (e.g., zinc, selenium, magnesium, iron, iodine, folate).

Stroke: When a vessel in the brain, which delivers blood to a defined region of the brain, is obstructed by a thrombus, the brain cells which depend on that vessel are in danger, because they do not obtain oxygen and nutrients any more. This is called an ischemic stroke. If the vessel ruptures, the brain cells will be damaged due to haemorrhage (bleeding). In addition, they do not obtain the necessary substrates any longer. In the prehospital setting, the cause of the stroke cannot be determined. It is of utmost importance, to diagnose the stroke rapidly and take the patient to the right hospital, one that has a stroke unit, immediately.

Aeronautical Glossary

Here, you will find short explanations to all aeronautical terms used in this book. A "=>" before a term within an explanation indicates that it is listed in the glossaries as well.

Air accident, quotation of the official definition:

"When the following terms are used in the Standards and Recommended practices for Aircraft Accident and Incident Investigation they have the following meaning:

Accident. An occurrence associated with the operation of an aircraft which takes place between the time any person boards the aircraft with the intention of flight until such time as all such persons have disembarked, in which:

a) a person is fatally or seriously injured as a result of

- being in the aircraft, or
- direct contact with any part of the aircraft, including parts which have become detached from the aircraft, or
- direct exposure to jet blast,

except when the injuries are from natural causes, self inflicted or inflicted by other persons, or when the injuries are to stowaways hiding outside the areas normally available to the passengers and crew: or

b) the aircraft sustains damage or structural failure which:

- adversely affects the structural strength, performance or flight characteristics of the aircraft, and
- would normally require major repair or replacement of the affected component,

except for engine failure or damage. when the damage is limited to the engine, its cowlings or accessories: or for damage limited to propellers, wing tips, antennas, tires, brakes, fairings, small dents or puncture holes in the aircraft skin: or

c) the aircraft is missing or is completely inaccessible.

Note I.– For statistical uniformity only, an injury resulting in death within thirty days of the date of the accident is classified as a fatal injury by ICAO.

Note 2.– An aircraft is considered to be missing when the official search has been terminated and the wreckage has not been located."

Source: International Standards and Recommended Practices, Aircraft Accident and Incident Investigation, Annex 13, to the Convention on International Civil Aviation, https://www.iprr.org/manuals/Annex13.html, most recently accessed: September 16th, 2023

Air traffic control (ATC): Either in the tower of an airport, or in the sections, which cover the airspace seemlessly, air traffic controllers guide the planes along their routes by assigning them headings and flight levels (certain altitudes) and giving them other directions. ATC has to make sure that planes are separated appropriately, and they also provide information, for instance, on weather conditions.

Cabin crew: The flight attendants play a decisive role in safety. They look at the passengers as they board the aircraft (Does this passenger seem fit to fly?), help in case of small injuries or minor discomfort, such as a headache. They know how to act in case of an emergency, in which they must cause the passengers to follow their instructions and prevent them from panicking.

Controlled flight into terrain (CFIT): Pilots of an airworthy aeroplane deviate unintentionally from their heading and altitude, for example, in adverse weather conditions, or close to an airport in a mountainous region. As a result, the aeroplane is flown into the surrounding terrain, an obstacle, or into the water.

Electronic centralised aircraft monitor (ECAM): It monitors many functions of the aeroplane and displays the results to the pilots. Furthermore, it detects malfunctions and provides information on what actions to take in order to solve the issues.

Flight crew: It usually consists of the captain, the first officer, sometimes a second officer, and a relief crew on longer flights to allow for rest periods. The pilot flying (PF) flies the plane (this might also be the first officer), whilst the pilot monitoring (PM) monitors the actions of the PF, as well as the progression of the flight. He or she also handles radio conversation and supports the PF (for instance, reading checklists). On earlier aircraft, there were also a flight engineer and a navigator.

Heterodyne: Pilots communicate with ATC using two-way VHF radios. On these, only one person can speak at a time as opposed to a telephone, on which both parties can speak simultaneously. If two pilots from different aircraft use their radios at the same time, the transmissions from these block each other out resulting in a garbled noise.

Incident, quotation of the official definition, see also => accident: "An occurrence, other than an accident, associated with the operation of an aircraft which affects or could affect the safety of operation." **Serious Incident:** "An incident involving circumstances indicating that an accident nearly occurred. Note 1.– The difference between an accident and a serious incident lies only in the result."

Knot: 1 knot equals 1.852km/h and 1.151 mph.

Line oriented safety audit (LOSA): Like => TEM, to which it is closely related, LOSA was developed as part of the sixth generation of => CRM. During routine flights (line operations), pilots are monitored in the cockpit by trained observers who collect data on how the pilots deal with => threats, => errors and => UASs. The pilots are not held accountable for their actions. In addition, the observers take notes of potential threats to safety and behaviours which are linked to => incidents and => accidents.

Maintenance resource management (MRM): As roughly 20% of air incidents and accidents are due to errors made during the maintenance of aircraft, MRM was created from CRM, adapting the principles of the latter to the peculiarities of the aircraft technicians´ workplaces in huge and noisy hangars.

PAN PAN PAN: The international signal which pilots declare to => ATC when they are in a hazardous situation in which they may need assistance quickly. The signal prompts ATC to prioritise this message.

Sterile cockpit rule: During phases of the flight with a high workload or in the middle of a potentially dangerous situation, the communication in the cockpit is solely about the tasks at hand and not about private issues. Also, activities, which have nothing to do with flying, are prohibited.

Uncontained engine rotor failure (UERF): In case of an UERF, the engine of an airliner not only malfunctions, but even disintegrates, and parts of it are catapulted out of its casing. These parts can hit the fuselage or endanger people, or any structure, on the ground.

Undesired aircraft state (UAS): A UAS is the result of an => error, and not a => threat. It reduces the safety margin. Examples include: wrong heading and altitude, or using the wrong taxiway.

Index